Max Pemberton is a doctor, journalist and writer. He works full time in the NHS in mental health and has spent many years working in drug addiction. He is a columnist for the *Daily Telegraph* and *Reader's Digest*, as well as a contributor to the *Mail On Sunday*. He has won several awards for his writing, including the Mind Journalist of the Year and the Royal College of Psychiatrists Public Educator of the Year award. He has also written three other books, including *Trust Me I'm a Junior Doctor*, which was serialised on Radio 4 Book of the Week. He lives and works in London.

Stop Smoking

with
CBT

The most powerful way
to beat your addiction

DR MAX PEMBERTON

Vermilion
LONDON

1 3 5 7 9 10 8 6 4 2

Vermilion, an imprint of Ebury Publishing,
20 Vauxhall Bridge Road,
London SW1V 2SA

Vermilion is part of the Penguin Random House group of companies
whose addresses can be found at global.penguinrandomhouse.com

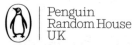

Copyright © Dr Max Pemberton 2014

Dr Max Pemberton has asserted his right to be identified as the author of this
Work in accordance with the Copyright, Designs and Patents Act 1988

First published by Vermilion in 2014

www.eburypublishing.co.uk

A CIP catalogue record for this book is available from the British Library

ISBN 9780091955120

Printed and bound by CPI Group (UK) Ltd, Croydon CR0 4YY

Penguin Random House is committed to a sustainable future for our
business, our readers and our planet. This book is made from
Forest Stewardship Council® certified paper.

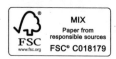

Contents

Introduction. 1

PART ONE: WHY PEOPLE SMOKE

1. First things first 15
2. An abusive relationship 22
3. Giving up. 26
4. Ex-smokers are the worst 28
5. Peer pressure and the first time. 31
6. Brainwashing 38

PART TWO: THE BASICS OF ADDICTION

7. The myth of nicotine addiction 43
8. Understanding the effects of nicotine 48
9. Getting to grips with addiction 57
10. Cravings. 62
11. The power of the mind. 66
12. Willpower 69
13. Life without smoke 71
14. Why do people keep smoking?. 73

PART THREE: YOUR THOUGHTS ABOUT SMOKING

15. The lies we tell ourselves. 79
16. Thinking errors. 89
17. Reasons to continue vs reasons to quit 94
18. The stages of change. 97

19. Getting stuck 101

20. Heroin 109

21. Ambivalence. 111

22. Desire. 113

23. Coping strategies 115

24. Cues. 118

25. Timeline. 121

26. Weight worries 128

27. Physical benefits of not smoking. 134

PART FOUR: ACTION

28. Preparing for action 141

29. Set a date 143

30. Detoxify your house. 148

31. Getting rid of smoking paraphernalia. 149

32. Reducing before stopping. 151

33. Tell a friend 153

34. Write a contract 155

35. Money talks 157

36. Nicotine replacement therapies or medications. 160

37. Avoiding triggers and breaking routines 165

38. When triggers remain. 168

39. Withdrawals. 170

40. Dealing with relapse. 176

41. Q&As 179

Conclusion: The best thing you've ever done 191

Resources 193

Acknowledgements. 194

Index 195

Introduction

STOP PANICKING

Before you start reading this book I want a quiet word. I know that you're probably quite scared right now, or at least a bit nervous. It's fine. Before I stopped smoking, I was petrified. The idea of reading a book on the subject would have made me physically sick. But I want you to relax, take a deep breath and stop panicking.

There is nothing scary inside this book. It is just a book. It can't make you do anything you don't want to. But the fact you've picked this book up and started reading suggests that, like all smokers out there, there is a part of you that longs to be free from it. All smokers live with a horrible tension between doing something they think they enjoy, and knowing that it is doing them tremendous, irreparable damage. This conflict creates all sorts of problems for smokers and is the source of much anguish. All this book will do, as long as you read it all and do exactly what I tell you, is help you change the way you think about smoking. The by-product of this is that you will no longer feel under the spell of nicotine and you will actually not want to smoke. You won't feel the need, and, what's more,

1

it will be one of the most exciting, exhilarating and thrilling things you'll ever do.

This book is not a lecture about why you shouldn't smoke or how evil it is or how it's going to kill you. What would be the point in that? There are thousands of articles and books and research papers that can tell you that – these days even the sides of cigarette packets themselves tell you how bad they are for you. There is not a single smoker who doesn't know the dangers of smoking and the damage it does to your body.

I'm a doctor and I smoked like a chimney, along with plenty of other doctors and nurses who know the risks in minute detail, and yet still continue to smoke. If explaining the risks to people worked, then there wouldn't be any smokers. What's the point in explaining it again? It's actually one of the things I hate most about doctors – the way they smugly sit there at their desk, with a shiny pen in their hand and a pot plant on their windowsill, and say, 'You should give up smoking; it's bad for you, you know,' as if all smokers are complete morons who have lived under a stone for the past five decades. I really doubt that a single person in the entire world has ever walked out of the surgery after a doctor has muttered those asinine words and thought, 'Well, I'd better stop then,' and ditched their cigarettes in the nearby bin. At best, all comments like that do is have the patient make a mental note to lie the next time they sit in front of the doctor. I lied to my GP for years about the fact that I smoked.

So, this book isn't going to lecture you or simply tell you things you already know that clearly haven't helped you. It is, however, going to go a little bit into the science of smoking and what happens when you inhale a cigarette. The reason for this is not to bamboozle you with information, but because knowing what is going on inside your body when you smoke and understanding how nicotine makes you addicted will take away some of the fear about stopping. You'll understand what withdrawal really is and have the proper science to hand. This is important because so much of what people say about smoking is just tripe, and some of it is even designed to stop you from stopping smoking. It's the lies we are told about smoking that prevent us from realising how easy it is to stop.

The thing to remember is that, unless someone has sat you down, strapped you into a chair, held your eyelids open with matchsticks and put this book in front of you, you're reading it because there is at least a part of you that wants to stop smoking – and you have listened to it, regardless of how quiet that voice was and is. So relax and indulge that voice a little bit. You have nothing to lose and, in fact, if you read the book and do everything it asks you to, you'll end up achieving something truly wonderful that you'll be unbelievably proud of.

THE TECHNIQUE

I have developed this stop-smoking programme using similar techniques to the ones doctors, psychologists and psychotherapists use on all sorts of patients who want to change their behaviour. They are used for a wide range of problems and conditions. I reasoned that if these techniques could change people who were feeling anxious or depressed, then surely they must be able to work in doing something as sensible and straightforward as stopping smoking.

The main techniques used are from a type of therapy known as 'cognitive behavioural therapy' – or CBT for short. You might have come across this term before, especially regarding it helping people overcome depression. However, if this term is new to you, then, in brief, CBT is a type of talking therapy that was first developed as a psychological treatment in the 1960s, and since then it has become one of the main methods used by doctors and psychologists for helping people with a range of psychological problems. It works by inviting the patient to examine aspects of their life that are causing them difficulties or problems and to challenge some of the unhelpful thoughts that they have and that are contributing to the problem. The aim of CBT is to help you change how you think about something – and therefore how you behave. I often describe it to patients as 'retraining' your brain how to think in a more helpful way.

CBT is used to treat a wide number of problems from depression, anxiety and panic attacks, through to other conditions like fatigue or pain. It's very good at helping you to make sense of a problem that you feel is overwhelming and that is making you feel 'stuck'. It does this by breaking things down into five main areas to help you see how the different aspects of the problem are connected and how they affect you. These areas are:

- A situation
- Thoughts
- Emotions

- Physical feelings
- Actions

How you think about a problem affects how you feel about it. Here's a diagram that is often used to explain this:

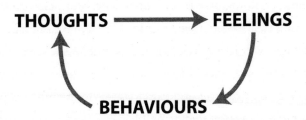

We can apply this to smoking. If you think that you'll never be able to stop smoking, or that you'll be miserable not smoking, or that it will be impossibly difficult, then you'll feel despondent and scared and depressed.

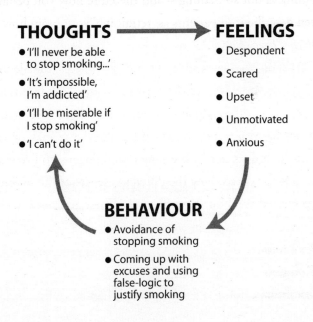

The solution to this is to avoid stopping smoking (and probably to light up a cigarette because you're stressed) and to tell yourself all sorts of things that will make you feel better about keeping smoking and avoiding the need to stop.

By tackling smoking in this way, it helps us to understand our thoughts about smoking and how this impacts on our behaviour. And by changing our thinking around smoking, it can help us change the behaviour.

There is another technique that I have also used in this book: motivational interviewing. This is usually used by doctors and therapists working with people addicted to drugs or alcohol. It aims to help the patient focus on their goal of abstinence by strengthening their own motivation for change and helping them commit to this. The key to this technique is to acknowledge that there are different stages of readiness for changing one's behaviour and that it is crucial to resolve any ambivalence towards making changes.

There is part of you that wants to stop smoking, or you wouldn't be reading this book. Motivational interviewing techniques can help you listen to this voice and realise that it's stronger and more powerful than the voice telling you to keep smoking.

HOW TO READ THIS BOOK

The book is separated into four main parts. Each one gently builds on the part before it and contains various chapters that will explore different aspects of smoking and the ways our minds keep us doing something we wished we didn't.

Interspersed throughout these chapters are exercises. They are not evenly spaced throughout the book because they arise naturally out of what is being discussed in a particular section. The exercises are integral to the programme and it's important that you do them, even if you can't see the point of them yet. They build on one another, as you will see as you progress through the book. Don't skip the exercises but also, don't just skim through the book looking for the exercises – without the groundwork in the text, they will be relatively meaningless.

Apart from that, how you choose to read this book is up to you. It might be that you've already made the decision to stop smoking and are eager to get it over and done with. That's fine. You can probably read the whole of this book quite easily in an afternoon. I don't want to be too prescriptive and stop you doing this – I've deliberately kept this book relatively short because I want those who aren't used to reading, or who don't have much time, to not feel overwhelmed by having a weighty tome to wade through. However, one thing that requires a longer amount of time is the exercises. One or two of them ask you to record your smoking habits over one whole day or more. Even if you finish reading the book before completing these exercises, you should still finish them before your actual quit date. Sometimes there's a tendency for people to want to rush things, and you might feel that the exercises requiring time and reflection are slowing you down. Please try to resist the temptation to skip these exercises. You're retraining your brain out of something that has held you in its grip for a long while, and this takes a bit of time.

If you want to read the book in one or two sittings, then by all means do, but mark the exercises that you haven't done and come back to them, reading the section of the book they relate to again to refresh your memory.

Alternatively, if you are more of a leisurely reader and just want to meander your way through, reading a bit here and there, that's fine, but do take care to read the book with some regularity so that the key messages don't get forgotten or lost between reading sessions.

No matter how you decide to read the book, please do the exercises. They're not here just to make the book look pretty. They are a fundamental part of the programme and are essential in helping to retrain your brain. From my experience, it usually takes people about one or two weeks to get through the book and do the exercises. Then they choose their stop date and stop smoking. If for some reason it doesn't work for you, then go back, reread the book and do the exercises again.

CAN THE BOOK BE USED WITH OTHER STOP-SMOKING TECHNIQUES?

There are various NHS programmes and support available to help you stop smoking, and many of them use techniques that are similar to the ones in this book. This is because they have a good evidence base and have been shown to work. Using this book doesn't mean you can't attend these sessions, or get support and help from your GP or pharmacist to stop smoking. As I'll discuss later on, using this book doesn't even mean you can't use nicotine gum or patches or take anti-smoking medications. This book is designed to help you change your thinking about why you smoke and therefore can happily sit alongside any other techniques you might choose.

I know that for some people the thought of going to the doctor or seeing a smoking-cessation counsellor at their GP surgery is very daunting and far too much like a commitment to stopping smoking. That's fine – this book is for you too as it will just gently invite you to think about your smoking in a different way from the safety and security of your own home.

GETTING STARTED

Before we get properly started, I need you to do some things first. Don't worry, this isn't at all as ominous as it sounds.

The first thing, if you don't already have some, is to go and buy some cigarettes. Now make the most of this – it isn't often that a doctor tells you to actually go and buy cigarettes. I don't want you to cut back while you're reading this book. There are bound to be times when certain topics might make you more anxious or you might get a desperate craving for cigarettes. That's fine. You're not failing in any way. Have a cigarette. All it means is we've touched on a nerve for you. It's useful to know, because it means that this is something you should focus on. If, for example, you start to get the craving for a cigarette when you're reading the section on social occasions, then it might be worth reading that part twice. You might find that, as we get further into the book, the desire to smoke gets less and less, and that's fine – don't force yourself to smoke, for goodness' sake. But, whenever you feel like it, spark up and puff away. I don't mind and neither should you.

The reason I say this is that I know how horrifying the prospect of not smoking is. The fact that you've picked up this book has probably increased your anxiety levels quite a bit already. If I now told you that you couldn't smoke, you'd probably either turn into a gibbering wreck or you'd simply stop reading, throw this book in the bin and light up.

The one exception to all this is if you have already stopped smoking but want some extra support around the psychological aspect of your addiction and are using the book for this. Obviously, don't start back up smoking again. You can still do all the exercises but, with the exercises that look specifically at when you smoke and the triggers for this, base them on when you used to smoke.

The key thing is, I'm never going to tell you to stop smoking. By the end of the book, you won't actually want to smoke. You'll close the book a non-smoker and wonder what all the fuss was about. You won't worry about cravings, or what to do with your hands, or how you'll get through social situations or stressful events or how you'll relax or keep calm or enjoy another meal or glass of wine. You'll see smoking for what it is: a trick of the mind that you fell for but that you've reprogrammed yourself out of. So don't worry. If you are worrying, you can have a cigarette now.

So go and get your cigarettes. Also, I want you to get a notepad and a pencil or pen. You should keep these by your side as you read the book, as you'll need them to do the exercises. I suggest you buy a notebook specifically for this and label it so it doesn't get filled with shopping lists or other notes.

You'll also need a diary or calendar and a box of matches. You don't need to keep these things with you the entire time, but you'll need them at various points, so it's worth being prepared.

Some of the chapters have homework (I know, it's like school, but console yourself that no one is going to steal your sandwiches or give you a wedgie, and there are certainly no quadratic equations). I do ask you to do the homework – the method I've developed is most effective if you do exactly as I ask. One final point about the homework though – I'm going to ask you to write some things down about how you feel and your thoughts. Now, this might be quite personal and I don't want you to feel embarrassed about what you write down, so don't show anyone else the homework, unless you really want to. It's important that you're as honest with yourself as possible, so if you think that anyone else seeing what you write down might hamper this, then keep it to yourself. You're doing this for yourself, not anyone else, and others should respect that.

So, you need cigarettes, a box of matches, something to write with, something to write on and your calendar or diary, if you have one. Easy.

PART ONE

WHY PEOPLE SMOKE

In this section we are going to start to explore some of the reasons why people first start smoking. While you might not think that the reasons you tried your first ever cigarette are important, the decision to do so has resulted in the current situation you are in, so it's important you revisit this and consider some of the thoughts that went with this behaviour. We will look at the idea of peer pressure and how the associations we have with smoking are developed long before we actually smoke.

1

First things first

I have a confession to make. The fact I'm writing this book has rather astounded me. I had pretty much given up on giving up smoking. I tried absolutely every possible way to give up. Patches, pills, gum, sprays, cold turkey, hypnosis. None of them worked. In fact, after trying some of them, I found I was smoking more than I was before. I've got no major axe to grind with any of these methods – with varying degrees of success, they help lots of people quit. But what I wanted to do was to remove my *desire* for cigarettes and I wasn't convinced that any of these ways actually did that. My greatest fear when I thought about giving up was that I would spend the rest of my life miserable because I couldn't smoke. I'd rather have died young as a smoker than live longer as a miserable ex-smoker. You're probably the same.

The thing is, I loved cigarettes. I mean, really loved them. I loved everything about them. I loved buying the packet and picking open the seal to the cellophane wrapping and opening the box for the first time. I loved opening the top and finding the paper lining neatly folded over the top of them and the slight resistance it gave as you pulled against the perforations. I loved the look of a full pack, the little white circles neatly arranged and looking up at me. I loved the sound of my lighter and the crackling of the tobacco as I lit the cigarette, and the burn of the first breath as it went down into my lungs. I loved the sigh as the smoke billowed out in a tight stream, unfurling and dissipating in rolling clouds. I was, to put it simply, in love with cigarettes.

Throughout my twenties I told myself that I would give up one day. One Day. That seemed reassuringly far away to prevent me panicking too much, but also definitive enough to fool myself into thinking I'd give up before it killed me. I set an arbitrary date, years ahead. When I'm 30, I decided. Yes, when I'm 30. That sounded like a good age. The kind of age that people grow up and stop doing silly things like smoking – because, deep down, I always knew that smoking was silly. Some would even say, stupid. But then 30 came and went, and nothing happened. It was several more years before I realised that, if I didn't make a concerted effort, I'd be smoking until I died. I started looking at people in their fifties and sixties who smoked. Would that be me one day?

I was in a muddle. I loved smoking, but I knew it was killing me. As a teenager I used to run the 1,500 kilometres at county level. I was quite good. But over the years I'd slowly come to notice that my fitness level was getting worse and worse. I'd get out of breath just thinking about running. I told myself I didn't care: 'Jogging is for people who are too stupid to work out how to hail a cab,' I said to myself and anyone else who was nearby. I still went to the gym regularly but stopped doing cardio and just did weights. I told myself it was because I wanted to look good naked and didn't care about fitness, but actually I knew it was because I couldn't face the idea of getting on a treadmill and seeing the damage I'd done to myself.

The more I thought about it, the more I realised it was perverse, but I couldn't help myself. That's what I kept saying: I can't help myself. Countless people nagged me to stop smoking. I even finished a relationship because the person hated me smoking. I was quite clear to him – I said, if you make me choose between you and cigarettes, I will choose cigarettes. He didn't believe me and made me choose. I cheerily waved him goodbye as I lit up.

I was a defiant smoker. Over the years of my smoking career the government imposed more and more restrictions on smoking. I wrote furious articles in the national press denouncing the moves as 'anti-libertarian' and 'health fascism'. I'd tried to stop a few times but had failed miserably. I'd tried every nicotine replacement therapy there was. Most helped me reduce my smoking for some time, cutting down from 20 a day to 10 for a while, but I missed not being able to smoke as many as I wanted and hated always counting and rationing myself, so I was soon back up to the usual amount. However, by then I was chewing gum or eating lozenges on top, so when I gave up using them I started smoking even more. I went from smoking 20 a day to 40 a day, thanks to gum. I was a nicotine junkie.

And then, one day, as I was sitting on a train on my way to work, I heard my thoughts out loud for the first time. My gran and aunt had just died from lung cancer, and this had brought on a new round of nagging from my mum about my smoking. And then there was the cough. At about this time, there was a government campaign saying that if you'd had a cough for a month, you should go to the GP to get it checked out as it might be cancer. I'd had my cough for five months, which my family had mentioned to me and, if I'm honest, I'd started to worry about.

And then, in a moment of horrifying clarity it occurred to me that even if it did turn out to be nothing, unless I decided to stop smoking, there was a high probability that at some point in my life I'd have a cough or some other symptom and that time it *would* be something serious, and I'd have cancer. For that brief moment I could imagine what it must be like to sit in front of a doctor and be given the horrible, earth-shattering news, and then having to walk out with the cars driving past and people sitting on benches, all going about their lives, totally oblivious. I'm sure you've had similar thoughts too – it's common for smokers to worry about this, but we've all got an incredible ability to push these thoughts out of our mind as soon as they appear, although deep within they often niggle. For the moment, I could hold on to the fact that I was young and it was highly unlikely to be anything sinister that was causing my cough, but in 20 years' time I wouldn't have my youth to hide behind. I still thought I loved smoking but I realised that I needed to have a good, hard think about my smoking and what I was going to do about it. I needed to make sure that I definitely loved it enough that I wouldn't mind dying for it.

Needless to say, I went to the GP and had a chest X-ray and it wasn't cancer. I lit up straight after that stressful doctor's appointment, but something in my head had changed. There had been a shift. I was beginning to question my relationship with cigarettes: was this love? Or was I a deluded fool?

It began to strike me that lots of the things I was hearing myself say were horribly similar to the things that I'd heard my patients say when I'd worked in a drug rehab clinic for people addicted to heroin and crack. I had heard every excuse under the sun to justify doing something that, to everyone else, was utterly bonkers, making them miserable and clearly killing them. I felt sick to the pit of my stomach. I was just like those heroin addicts I worked with. I was making excuses.

I realised I had a choice. You have a choice too. Every time you light up a cigarette you are making a choice to smoke. It might not feel like a choice – it might feel like you are compelled to light up – or you might feel like it's a choice you *want* to make. But, just like my patients who were addicted to drugs, I came to realise that the things I thought I was basing my choices on were in fact false logic.

I realised, also, that smoking is rather like self-harm. I had worked with many people who chose to physically harm themselves. For such troubled people the act of, for example, cutting themselves is a release – a way of coping with life. It's also a very flawed coping strategy: while it may momentarily give some sense of control, in reality it clearly doesn't. There's nothing inherent in cutting yourself that changes the fact you don't have the money for the electricity bill, for example. The same is true for smoking – you might think, for example, that smoking helps you relax, but you'll see later how this isn't the case.

In fact, smoking and self-harming share a number of similarities. They both rely on the mind falsely associating a behaviour with relief and pleasure, and of alleviating stress and anxiety, yet are both ultimately damaging. And, despite the fact that this is obvious, people still partake in these activities.

Once people have fallen into this compulsive behaviour, it's very difficult for them to stop. Difficult, but not impossible. In fact, in the unit where I worked, many of the patients were undergoing CBT or versions of this. It struck me that some of the techniques that these patients used to curb the urge they had to deal with their problems by self-harming could be applied to smoking. Shouldn't I perhaps apply some of the thinking I was trying to get my patients to engage with to myself?

I tried to think about my behaviour objectively. I knew that if an alien came down and watched what I did repeatedly during the day – lit up something that I knew was poisonous and purposefully put it inside my body – they would think I was stark staring mad. At that moment, something in my head clicked. If I'd been at work and this had been with a patient, this would be called a cognitive shift: I'd shifted the way I thought about something. My entire view had changed. I realised I was in a hateful, harmful relationship that was killing me, that I got nothing from and yet took so much from me. I needed to fall out of love with cigarettes. I knew that this is what I wanted to achieve, but I knew I'd have to work in order to actually do it.

You might have had a similar experience that has led you to pick up this book. Or you might just be looking for the inspiration to help you make the leap to wanting to quit. Either way, you are likely to feel somewhat anxious and quite sad at the prospect of stopping something that, at the moment, you probably think gives you pleasure. However, over the course of the book, you'll learn how to challenge the thinking that underpins this belief.

We often think about stopping smoking as a single event – the actual stopping. But this isn't the case. Stopping smoking is a process. It begins with starting to question the behaviour – as had happened to me sitting on the train, and will happen to you reading through this book. When you do this, you'll discover that it's perfectly possible to fall out of love with smoking and see it for what it really is: a trap that you've fallen into but that you can set yourself free from.

2
An abusive relationship

I want you to view smoking as a relationship. This analogy is useful because it shows you how people can change their view about things. Let me explain.

Imagine you are in the first throes of a relationship. At the beginning everything is hunky-dory. You take a few tentative steps, go on some dates, maybe sleep with them (it's fine, I'm not your mother – I'm not judging you). Before you know it, you're in a full-blown relationship. Wow, you think, how did that happen? You made a choice to be with that person, but perhaps you didn't really appreciate the commitment you were making to this one person who, you realise, maybe you didn't know quite as well as you thought you did. Still, it's something to do and they provide you with someone to go to the cinema with, plus sharing a bed saves on heating costs, and things could be worse, right? Now obviously I'm not talking about the love of your life here. This is one of those relationships that isn't quite right – one of the ones that doesn't make it.

Eventually, the relationship ends and – this is the key bit – after you've moped about for a bit, you look back on that relationship and see it precisely for what it was: something that, actually, was a bit rubbish. The idea of dating that person again makes you recoil in horror. You have, essentially, fallen out of love with them. You don't even hate them (hate is too similar to love) – you're just indifferent to them with an undertone of slight disbelief that you ever thought they were right for you. You're gently puzzled that you could ever have convinced yourself that all their annoying habits and personality flaws didn't bother you. And, of course, this had often been glaringly obvious to anyone on the outside, looking in on your relationship, but you had ignored them.

Smoking is just the same. Think of all those people who have tried to tell you to stop smoking: the worried shakes of the heads, the imploring looks of 'please give up soon', the gentle questioning about when you are going to kick the habit. But both you and I know that to the smoker – just as to the person who is in a bad relationship – these interventions rarely work. Changing the way we think about something usually takes a lot more work than the odd chat. In fact, with smoking, the more people tell you not to do it, the more you think, 'Screw you, I'll do what I want!' I'm right, aren't I?

How is it possible that smokers can love something that is so patently bad for them – that, really, gives them nothing in return for their devotion to it? The problem here is that people confuse being 'in love' with being 'in need'. Smokers think they love cigarettes and that it gives them pleasure because it's what we have been conditioned to believe. It's all part of the enormous con trick that makes up smoking. We think we love cigarettes but actually they give us nothing and we confuse loving them with needing them. We need them because we're addicted to the drug they contain: nicotine. That is all.

But even if you are convinced that you really do love cigarettes – as I was – as past relationships show, it's perfectly possible to fall out of love with something and to not miss it in the slightest. You can look back on the past when you were smoking with bemusement at how you could have ever thought it was a good idea. We'll explore this idea in more detail later, but, for the time being, I want you to just keep this in your mind:

- No matter how much you think you love something now, it is possible to fall out of love.
- People who no longer love something don't miss it.
- Smokers love something that doesn't love them back. They are in a relationship that is worse than abusive; it's deadly.

EXERCISE 1: THE REASONS YOU SMOKE

With all this in mind, the first thing I want you to do is to write a list of what you love about cigarettes. It doesn't matter how daft some of the things are or how superficial. It's important that you start to examine what you think cigarettes give to you. Maybe you think they make you feel more confident or more relaxed. The only rule to this list is that you're not allowed to simply write that you enjoy them or love them: I want you to write why. What do you think you get from smoking – after all, it must give you something, otherwise why do it? What are the positive things that smoking makes you feel?

For me, it was feeling rebellious and naughty; I felt it helped me in social situations, helped me relax and helped me focus. These were the things that I told myself smoking gave me. These were the things at the root of my apparent love for cigarettes, and, most importantly, it was because of these things that I was convinced I wouldn't be able to stop smoking.

So make your list of reasons to continue smoking. You can spend some time on this and really think about it. You can add things to the list as you think of them. Remember, this list is just for you, so don't be inhibited about what you write down. Keep it somewhere safe and we'll come back to it later.

3
Giving up

The purpose of this book is not to get you to give up smoking. If you give up smoking there is a fair chance that you will spend months, if not years, longing for a cigarette. It will torment you, and, let's be honest, while you might live longer because you're not smoking, you might wonder what's the point if you're always miserable about the fact you're not smoking. No, this book isn't going to help you *give up* smoking because you are not going to give anything up. *Giving up* suggests that you are denying yourself something. When you stop smoking you are absolutely not denying yourself anything because smoking gives you absolutely nothing. I know that you've just made a list of the things you think that smoking gives you, but over the course of this book, you'll learn to view this list differently.

So from now on, I don't want you to use the term 'giving up' but instead, to use the terms stopping or quitting. This is important because on an unconscious level we are programmed to believe that smoking gives us something – otherwise why would we do it? – when in fact the opposite is true.

This is a vital point so I'm going to repeat it: you are not going to give up smoking because you are not giving anything meaningful up. Giving something up suggests that you are denying yourself something, and you are not. You are not denying yourself anything by not smoking. Smoking does not give you anything. Say it back to yourself. Go on.

So, what this book is about is stopping smoking. It's a behaviour you do and you are going to stop it. It's that simple.

4
Ex-smokers are the worst

The idea that ex-smokers are 'the worst' is often true, and there's a psychological explanation for this, which I'll explain in a minute. This book will not make you an *ex-smoker*. It will make you a *non-smoker*. As with 'giving up', this sounds like semantics, but it's important. An ex-smoker is someone that still, deep down, wants to smoke. They are defined by something they used to do. An ex-smoker carries the fact they used to smoke with them like a weight around their neck, dragging them down.

One of two things happens to the ex-smoker. In the first instance, they spend the rest of their lives miserable and wishing they could smoke, tortured by pangs every time they think about smoking or are near smokers. This is nothing to do with physical addiction to cigarettes (which is over remarkably quickly, as we'll cover later) but the fact that they remain psychologically addicted to them. Ex-smokers often relapse because the torment of wanting to do something so much and not being able to is stronger than the desire of living a longer, healthier life. This anguished state is awful

– and precisely what I didn't want for myself and what I don't want for you.

The alternative group of ex-smokers love cigarettes but they know that they shouldn't, and so they take the opposite stance and openly condemn smokers and smoking. This sounds like a complicated trick for the mind to play but it's actually a very common mechanism that the mind employs to deal with conflicts. Psychologists call this tactic 'reaction formation', which basically means that unacceptable, anxiety-causing emotions or impulses (in the case of ex-smokers, 'I love cigarettes and wish I could still smoke') are masked by adopting an exaggerated version of the *opposite* emotion or impulse. Examples of this are all around and it's the basis of the phrase 'the lady doth protest too much'. A person who hates a work colleague may be excessively nice towards them, for example. People who make a big deal of being heterosexual and are openly homophobic often turn out to be having same-sex attractions themselves. And so on.

In the case of smoking, the ex-smoker is so eaten up by the deep-seated wish to smoke, which they are desperately trying to bury and ignore, that they take the opposite position. They are the nightmare person at a party who turns their nose up at the smokers, who loudly proclaims how disgusting they think smoking is and coughs dramatically and moves away, usually shaking their head.

You might argue that, well, at least the ex-smoker isn't smoking and this is a good thing. Sure, this is true. But there are two things that worry me about this. Firstly, the ex-smoker can be a pain to be around, especially at a party. They put smokers off from quitting because they look at the ex-smoker and think, 'I never want to be such a boring killjoy,' and they also look at their friends who smoke and think, 'Well, I'll never be able to be friends with them if I quit and they keep smoking.' We are naturally social animals and the thought of having to get rid of all your friends because you've given up smoking isn't going to be appealing. Secondly, I hate the idea that someone is beating themselves up – even if it is deep in their unconscious mind – about smoking because, really, not smoking is no big deal. It's nothing.

So, this book will not make you an ex-smoker, it will make you a *non-smoker*. Make sure you use this phrase to describe yourself when you stop smoking. After reading this book, you will no longer be defined by smoking – either doing it or not doing it – you will be entirely free from cigarettes and that means you no longer have to define yourself in relation to them. You'll be free and, the best bit, you won't be one of those awful tedious ex-smokers at the party.

5
Peer pressure and the first time

I first started smoking as a teenager. I remember it very clearly. We're always told that people start smoking because of peer pressure, and this immediately conjures up images of some pale, puny kid surrounded by a gang of older kids wearing leather jackets and sunglasses looking down at him and sneering. Of course, peer pressure doesn't really work like that (unless you inhabit some strange world where everyone looks like an extra from the film *Grease*). It's a far more subtle, insidious process. The gang goading you on to try it are in your head, rather than in the playground. It's that niggling curiosity: 'Other people are doing it and seem to like it, so there must be something in it for me.' Even more intoxicating and alluring – 'It's something adults do and don't want me to do.'

As we're going to find out, it's what goes on in your head that really matters with smoking (and so many things in life). This is how it was with me – there were no cigarette-pushing oiks goading me to try it, just that small voice in my head suggesting that I must be missing out on something and that if I smoked I'd be one of the cool kids. It was a small voice but, boy, it was powerful.

I was 14 and in an art class and it suddenly struck me: I could smoke. In fact, I *should* smoke, I concluded. That's what cool kids did, wasn't it, and I wanted to be cool, didn't I? I remember going over to my friend Andrew Swartfigure, who was doing something creative with clay – or he might have been trying to peer up a girl's skirt, I can't actually remember – and saying to him, 'Hey, Andrew, why don't we buy a packet of cigarettes and smoke them?' It was as simple as that.

A few days later, on a Saturday afternoon, he bought 10 Silk Cut and a box of matches from a newsagent while I waited around the corner trying not to look as though I was waiting round a corner for someone who was buying cigarettes for me. Then we sat in the park and lit one. We both looked at it for a while until it occurred to one of us that perhaps the one thing less cool than not smoking at all was not smoking while holding a lit cigarette and instead just staring at it. So I took a puff and, having heard that people always choke the first time, deliberately didn't inhale but just let the plumes of smoke drift out of my mouth. Cooool! Andrew did the same. We were smoking! After doing this a few more times Andrew had to go home so we went our separate ways and I bought a dozen packets of mints, which I chewed on the way home. I spent most of the next day on the toilet because the mints had some sweetener that in ludicrously high doses acted as a laxative, but that's by the by. I'd had my first cigarette and I liked it. Actually, I didn't like the cigarette at that point – I just liked the *idea* that I had smoked. So then, periodically when Andrew and I met up on a Saturday, we'd smoke a cigarette or two together while loitering about on the swings in the local park.

God, we felt so cool. In retrospect, of course, this was the mid-1990s and Andrew and I were both wearing shell suits, so we most certainly weren't that cool at all. But we felt cool. And that, incidentally, is really the crux of this book. Smoking itself isn't about the nicotine; it's about feelings. Part of what keeps us smoking is that we learn to associate it with all sorts of feelings that act as a perpetuator for the behaviour: fear, anxiety, boredom, stress, fitting in, wanting to be cool. We'll deal with all this later on, but you can see already how little old me at the tender age of 14 had, in some way, already learned to associate smoking with being cool, and so I started what was to become a nearly two-decade love affair.

It's quite possible that how I got started is quite similar – at least in a few key bits – to you, and it's important that you too think about why and how you started smoking. The legacy of that decision is with you now. You never thought you'd get addicted; it was just experimenting; you thought it would be cool; it was naughty and exciting and something to do, for example. But because of a series of quite possibly unrelated events you ended up in a situation whereby you had access to cigarettes, were able to try them and then, having tried them, to keep smoking them enough that you became addicted.

The other thing I want you to realise from reading my story is how, even before I had tried a cigarette, I had very clear, vivid notions about smoking and the sorts of people that smoked, and this helped to prompt me into trying it. These emotionally charged associations are not coincidence: they are part of an enormous, complex, far-reaching industry that had been tapping me on the shoulder for years before I ever thought about actually trying a cigarette. I guarantee that when you look back over your own story about trying cigarettes, you'll have similar associations with smoking: it's cool, it's naughty, it's rebellious or it's sophisticated.

Even though the tobacco industry can no longer advertise in many countries, the language of cigarettes still persists. It was carefully constructed for decades by the companies that pushed them, and one of the things that made the language they used so hard to resist was that it was based, at least in part, on truth. For youngsters, smoking is naughty and rebellious and exciting, precisely because their parents and adults don't want them to do it. This makes it all the more appealing. The types of people who smoke, as we'll see later, tend to be the types of people we want to be. All the tobacco industry had to do was ensure that we were exposed to all this enough times that we started to see it for ourselves. The associations with smoking and rebelliousness, excitement and naughtiness are still present today and it's the reason that, even without the help of film stars like James Dean, youngsters still smoke.

Stopping smoking is about change. This is partly why it's so scary. For many, many smokers, they think smoking is part of who they are. I know I did and you probably do too. I allowed it to define me: I was the naughty doctor who smoked, the maverick. I liked the idea I did something unexpected like smoking when I was supposed to know better; I was being contrary. Smoking for me was two fingers up to the establishment that I found myself entering, and yet didn't really feel I related to when I began medical school. The thought of stopping smoking horrified me because I genuinely couldn't believe that I'd be the same person afterwards. I didn't want to change. Of course, the reality is that when you stop smoking nothing actually changes; you're exactly the same person, you just don't smoke. But still we hold on to the fact that in some way smoking is part of us and underpins who we are as people. This thinking has its roots right back at the beginning of our relationship with cigarettes.

EXERCISE 2: YOUR SMOKING STORY

In this second exercise, I want you to spend some time thinking about yourself as a smoker. To do this, I want you to write your own story about your first experience of cigarettes in your notepad, much in the same way that I did just now. Don't worry if you don't think you're very good at writing or your spelling isn't very good. No one else is ever going to read this, so just write it however you want to. It's not the writing that's important – it's thinking about how your relationship with cigarettes developed. I want you to transport yourself back in time and remember *why* you tried your first cigarette. Ask yourself what it felt like – I don't just mean the actual act of smoking, I mean what it felt like *to be* smoking. Grown up? Cool? Sophisticated? This episode in your life is of vital importance because it set something in motion that you're still dealing with now. It's had a dramatic, costly and divisive impact on your life. You can't hope to move forward unless you've properly examined when this all started.

If you're not sure how to begin your story, then remember, you're not writing *War and Peace*. Don't allow yourself to get stuck because you're aiming for literary perfection. If it helps, you can write it as a letter to your younger self who has just tried their first cigarette. Write it as though you are explaining to them what happened after that moment when they had their first puff, telling them what was going through their mind and what it led on to.

Once you've described your first cigarette, I want you to think about the lead-up to you becoming addicted. These feelings are important because, even if you had them years ago, they are still there and still underpin your behaviour – even if you don't realise it. Ask yourself these questions:

1. What did you associate with smoking?
2. What made you keep trying to smoke?
3. Do you have romantic or exciting memories attached to it?

Include this in your account or letter. You can write all the good memories you have of smoking – the holidays, staying up late drinking wine with friends or whatever. The key to this is to be honest. You might not have any positive associations with smoking – you might hate it and wish you could be free of the blasted cigarettes. That's fine. But at some point in your life this wasn't the case, and I want you to try to get in touch with those memories and write them down. There's no right or wrong thing to write; it's about how you felt, the associations you made in your mind with smoking and how that impacted on your decision to become a smoker.

Spend some time writing your account. Now I want you to put it away and read it the next day. But when you read it, I want you to try to mentally detach yourself from it, so that you're not reading your own account, but someone else's. Think carefully about what you've written and try to spot the tricks that your mind was playing on you. For example, you thought it made you feel cool and grown up at the time, but do you now think you were that cool and grown up?

6
Brainwashing

Psychological experiments have shown that the average smoker tends to be an extrovert. Of course, there are exceptions to this, but on average, studies have shown that people who smoke have a certain type of personality. They tend to be greater risk takers, more daring, more rebellious and more defiant than those who've never smoked. They also tend to be more sexualised – reporting a higher-than-average need for sex – and studies have shown that younger people who smoke are also less likely to be virgins. Now, there's a whole host of complex social and psychological reasons for this, but can you think, from a marketing perspective, who could be better adverts for your product? It's a dream come true for any company to have their product associated with sexy, naughty, rebellious people, and this is exactly what the tobacco industry has. All it's had to do is make sure that the appropriate people – film stars, musicians, artists – are photographed and filmed smoking and that acts as the perfect advertising for them. Of course, what we fail to realise is that it's not actually smoking that's cool, it's the people, who happen to smoke, that are cool. But in our minds we get all this confused and we associate the object (cigarette) with the person's attributes (coolness, sophistication). This phenomenon is well known and indeed is utilised by other industries. The entire fashion industry is based on this – it's not the design label that is sexy, it's the attractive person modelling the clothes. But people buy the clothes because they think this will therefore make them sexy too. It's the same with smoking.

The fact that fusty, boring old parents tell youngsters not to smoke only makes it all the more appealing. This is in no way a defence of smoking or to say that parents shouldn't try to dissuade their kids from smoking. It's just important for you to realise that part of the brainwashing that's gone on in your head about smoking was there long before you smoked. It was building up slowly, insidiously, when you were going about your everyday life and just happened to watch a film where the hero (or anti-hero) was a smoker. Understand that you have been indoctrinated into making associations with smoking. These are what made it appealing to begin with and will, to a greater or lesser extent, still be there even now. So, think about your own story – about how, when and why you started smoking. Think about the language you associate with smoking, then and also now. Think about all the false associations and thoughts you had about smoking that meant you tried it and got hooked.

PART TWO

THE BASICS OF ADDICTION

In this section we're going to look at some of the basic science of smoking. We'll see why cigarettes are addictive, what happens when you smoke, how you become addicted and the truth about cravings, as well as the role the mind plays in all this. We're also going to explore the idea of willpower and why people keep smoking, even though they wish they didn't.

7

The myth of nicotine addiction

Smoking is one great big fat scam. Everything to do with it. We've just seen how we incorrectly assign to smoking all sorts of appealing characteristics and how this was carefully manipulated by the tobacco industry because it was entirely to its advantage to perpetuate the association between its products and being cool or sophisticated.

But this goes much further. From why you think you smoke, to how hard it is to give up, there are big, powerful, vocal groups and organisations with vested interests in perpetuating lies about it. We've all been brainwashed, and actually the knack to stopping smoking is to understand the lies we've all swallowed, including many in the medical profession.

The difficult bit about smoking is changing the way we think about it, rather than the physical withdrawal of nicotine. But what happens with smoking is that all these myths, all these lies and half-truths and misrepresentations of the truth, combine in our minds to create this horrible, awful, insurmountable thing – this grotesque ogre that we think we're not strong enough to tackle on our own. It's fear that stops people from giving up smoking, but, really, what is this fear of? No one dies from 'not smoking'.

There are many myths about smoking, but the most noxious, the most dangerous, is that it's terribly difficult to give up. I've even had patients relay to me in hushed, horrified whispers, that nicotine is the most addictive drug in the world. For a while I even believed this myself. It's the sort of thing that sounds like it should be true. However, this is complete, utter, unadulterated rubbish. Don't believe it for one moment.

There are two large, very powerful and unimaginably wealthy groups who have a significant vested interest in trying to perpetuate this lie. The first, of course, is the tobacco industry. Years ago, when people first began to question the safety of tobacco, it denied that it was addictive. But since then, faced with a wealth of research, while not exactly openly admitting it, it has stopped denying it. But, interestingly, analysis of cigarettes shows that the level of nicotine has been slowly creeping up in a direct relationship to the amount of people giving up. Of course, it's not that increasing the amount of nicotine is responsible for people giving up. It's more likely, as some researchers have suggested, that the level of nicotine delivered by each cigarette is increased in the hope it will stem the tide of people stopping. It will make it harder to quit.

Now, if nicotine was so addictive, why would the companies increase the amount of it in their product? Surely they wouldn't need to. Once someone is addicted to heroin, you don't need to increase the level of heroin they take to keep them addicted. No, the reality is that nicotine, as a drug, is not very effective at being addictive. Nicotine addiction is so weak that it doesn't wake you up when you're asleep. I can assure you, this isn't the case with alcohol or heroin addiction.

But the twist here is that, while they're never going to actively promote the notion that smoking is incredibly addictive, the tobacco industry is happy to allow the lie to be perpetuated because it makes those who are already hooked scared. And being scared means you are less likely to give up. And that means more customers.

The other group who want to keep you believing that cigarettes have this unnatural, almost magical, hold on you is the pharmaceutical industry. Now, I'm not some nutty tree-hugging Marxist who thinks that the pharmaceutical industry is filled with the most evil people on the planet and that it is solely responsible for all the ills of the world. I prescribe medicines every working day of my life. I'm acutely aware of the contribution that the pharmaceutical industry has made in the development of medicine and the eradication of diseases. I'm aware that through its innovation it alleviates suffering all over the world. However, it would be a bit daft of us not to look critically at it from time to time. The pharmaceutical industry has a vested interest in making sure that we all remain in fear of cigarettes because, as it knows only too well, where there's fear, there's money to be made. And, let's face it, pharmaceutical companies, just like any other company, are interested in making profits. That's how they work; they're not making products just for the fun of it.

It might come as a surprise to know that nicotine replacement therapy has been around for decades. In fact, pretty much as soon as the public became aware of the link between smoking and cancer, some clever boffin in a pharmaceutical company thought of the idea of creating a product that would help people stop smoking. It didn't take long and, within a few years, nicotine gum was being marketed as the quick-fix solution for those wanting to give up painlessly. If you're going to sell a product, you need a market and, if there isn't one already there, you have to make it. So, they set about telling the world how difficult it was to give up and that we all needed help. Ker-ching!

So we're bombarded with adverts and information telling us how difficult the task ahead of us is going to be and that we're going to fail if we don't use their products, and it never even occurs to us that the reason we're being told this is because people will make money out of it. We never think to question it. And the medical establishment have mostly swallowed it too. If you go to the doctor and say you want to stop smoking, they don't ever sit back in their chair and say, 'Go on then, it's actually not that difficult. You just need to change the thinking patterns that have become entrenched in your mind and it will be a doddle,' do they? No, they pick up their pen (which is probably advertising some nicotine gum) and write you a prescription for a nicotine replacement therapy.

Is this so bad? Well, I have one fundamental issue with the whole nicotine replacement industry and it's this: trying to quit by *just* using nicotine replacement therapy risks creating ex-smokers, because it doesn't deal with the deep-down psychological desire to smoke. All it does is deal with the addiction and, as we've just touched on, the physical addiction towards nicotine is actually very mild and not nearly as bad as you'd imagine. It's the *psychological* addiction that's the tricky bit, and this is precisely the part of smoking that nicotine replacement therapy doesn't tackle. So, if you're going to use nicotine replacement products, it's important that you also look to deal with the psychological side of your addiction.

Now I don't want you to run away with the idea that you're not addicted to nicotine. You are. I was too. All smokers are. That's why they smoke. What is important to realise is that this addiction is not as strong and troublesome and difficult to overcome as people have been telling you. You might not believe me now, but I promise you that is the case. By the time you have finished this book, you'll actually look forward to stopping smoking and you'll view the tiny, pathetic pangs of withdrawal as something to celebrate because it means you're ridding yourself of your addiction.

EXERCISE 3: REASONS TO CONTINUE SMOKING

I want you to write down a list of all the things that prevent you from stopping smoking. This might be harder than it sounds. Smoking is something we can do without really thinking about it most of the time, and it's easy for us to create myths and illusions around why we should keep doing it.

What is it that truly stops you from stopping? What is it that scares you? Write down your list, and, as always, you can add to it later as things occur to you. These are your reasons NOT to quit, or 'reasons to continue'.

8

Understanding the effects of nicotine

Why do we get addicted to smoking when we don't get addicted to, say, bananas, or courgettes or rice? Actually the reason that some substances are addictive and others aren't is down to a quirk of nature to do with basic biology.

It is worth spending some time understanding this because, when you're armed with the knowledge of what is happening to your body when you smoke, the whole process of quitting is demystified and you can see how breathtakingly simple and straightforward it is.

When you light a cigarette and inhale, the smoke is pulled down into your lungs. In the smoke are thousands of vaporised chemicals that were in the tobacco and various other chemicals that have been added to the tobacco to make it burn evenly and so on. Inhaling a chemical is a very effective way of getting it into your bloodstream, because the lung has a rich supply of blood. The lungs consist of several million tiny bulbs called alveoli. When you look at them under a microscope, they look a bit like a bunch of grapes, but when viewed with the naked eye they give the lung its spongy appearance. The point of these alveoli is to give the lung a very large surface area, which means that things can be absorbed very quickly. In fact, thanks to the alveoli, the total surface area of the lungs is equivalent to that of a tennis court. When the lungs expand they pull air into them and down, through all the tubes, into the alveoli. Here, oxygen from the freshly inhaled air is rapidly absorbed into the bloodstream and is then pumped around the body.

When a person inhales from a cigarette, that air brought down into the lungs is combined with all the chemicals from the smoke, and these too are absorbed into the bloodstream. In the smoke is tar, which is a sticky residue and bad for the lungs. There are also thousands of other chemicals in the smoke (including things like arsenic and various other poisons), but it's the nicotine – and only the nicotine – that's really important in becoming physically addicted to smoking. Within one second of inhaling cigarette smoke, the chemicals have been absorbed and are on their way to the brain. It's far quicker and more effective than swallowing or even absorbing it through the mouth, which is why many people complain that nicotine replacement therapy such as nicotine gum doesn't relieve the cravings in the same way as smoking does. So the key thing to realise here is that cigarettes are simply a device for delivering nicotine to the brain, in the same way that a margarita is a device for delivering alcohol to the brain.

However, unlike a margarita, cigarettes are actually quite unpleasant for the body. While manufacturers try to tell us we enjoy the 'taste' of them, actually, think back to that first cigarette you had – they taste foul. It's one of the world's greatest ironies that cigarette manufacturers have tried to sell us a product that tastes disgusting by marketing the taste! They use words like 'mild' and 'smooth' to try to get us to buy into the idea that the taste is nice. It's not. One of the side effects of smoking is that it kills off some of the taste buds on the tongue, as well as the sense of smell, so that, over time, we simply can't taste and smell quite how foul it is.

So, once the nicotine is in the blood and the blood has made its way to the brain, the interesting stuff starts to happen. The reason nicotine is addictive is because, by a quirk of nature, there is a receptor in the brain which nicotine can latch on to. A receptor is a protein that sits on the outside of a cell and, when activated, creates a chemical reaction inside the cell. It's like a lock that needs a specific key to activate it. Each cell has thousands of different receptors on its surface, each controlling different processes. Now, this quirk of nature means that nicotine happens to fit into a certain receptor.

The body didn't design it like this – it's just fluke – but it fits so neatly that scientists sometimes call it a nicotine receptor – or nicotinic acetylcholine receptor, to give it its full name. I've drawn a picture below to show you what I mean. It also shows you that I clearly should have paid more attention to my art teacher and less time talking to Andrew Swartfigure about smoking:

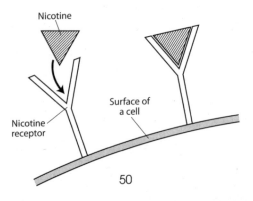

The fact there is a receptor for nicotine to latch on to is important for several reasons. The first is that the nicotine receptor happens to be all over the cells of the brain – in particular, the bits of the brain to do with feeling reward. So, when nicotine latches on to one of these receptors, it throws the switch that releases certain chemicals, such as dopamine, which, in this part of the brain, makes us feel satisfied, happy and relaxed. There are actually nicotine receptors all over the body but they are very slightly different in shape, so nicotine fits better to the ones in the brain than anywhere else. Because of its affinity for the receptors in this part of our brain, we quickly learn to associate inhaling smoke with obtaining a sense of reward. Of course, it's just a molecule of nicotine interacting with a receptor, which isn't really rewarding or satisfying for us in any meaningful sense, but it makes us *feel* rewarded and satisfied.

The second reason this is important is that over time, as you continue to smoke the occasional cigarette, the nicotine receptors start to notice that there is a lot of this nicotine chemical floating around and that it seems to really like attaching to it. It's then that the body does something very clever but also something that will cause untold misery later on. It starts to make more nicotine receptors. And more. And more. The biological term for this is 'receptor up-regulation' and the practical implications are that all of these receptors expect to be stimulated by nicotine. I think of them as lots of little baby birds, sitting in a nest with their beaks wide open, waiting for food. They continue to chirp loudly until they are fed. While one little bird is easy to ignore, a whole nest is harder. In the same way, while each receptor on its own doesn't pose too much of a problem, when there are lots of them, it creates the kind of noise that the brain can't ignore. It's these receptors shouting out to be filled with nicotine that is actually the basis of addiction. It's the empty receptors, calling out to be filled with a nicotine molecule that makes us spark up time and time again. When they're empty and haven't been stimulated for a while, this is what we term withdrawal.

The good news is that, when we stop stimulating the receptors with nicotine for long enough, the cells stop making them and actually start getting rid of the excess. This is called 'receptor down-regulation', and it means that, after quitting, eventually we'll have the normal amount of receptors and will have no more cravings. This dying back of the receptors starts a few days after you stop smoking, and the number is back to normal after a few months. If you can get past the first few days without smoking, then your body already reduces the receptors for nicotine in your brain and, as their number decreases, so will your cravings. For each minute you abstain from a cigarette, thousands of the receptors die off and you're one step closer to being free of your addiction.

There is one final reason why the receptors are important for us in understanding stopping smoking. We've all come across those people at parties or wedding receptions who, late at night and usually after a few drinks, will wander over to the smokers and ask for a cigarette. Often people will hand one over, a little bemused, saying that they didn't know that person smoked. 'Oh, I don't really,' and they then usually give some qualifier, such as only at weekends, or only after they've been drinking, or when their partner isn't there. For a long time, these people were a tantalising anomaly to me. I longed to be one of those people. I remember a friend's mum who used to keep a packet of 10 Silk Cut in the cutlery drawer and would smoke a cigarette once every few weeks – just when she felt like it. This was the kind of smoker I wanted to be. It would mean that I didn't *have* to smoke unless I wanted to; that I could reduce the frequency I did it to the extent that it would pose little risk to my health – that smoking would become something enjoyable again: a treat.

This thinking is flawed for several reasons, not least that, really, smoking is not enjoyable at all, we just think it is. But, putting this aside, I think many smokers would be very happy if they too could get to this sort of state – the very occasional, take-it-or-leave-it, once-in-a-blue-moon-when-I-feel-like-it smoker. I've got some bad news for you: it's never going to happen like that for you. And the reason for this is thanks to those pesky receptors, and I'll tell you why.

The other twist to the receptor story is that they vary in their shape very slightly from person to person. How well the nicotine can fit into the receptors depends on genetics, and I may as well break the news to you now: you drew the short straw. I did too. That's why I smoked and it's why you smoke.

Nicotine is, essentially, a poison. When we inhale smoke we're engaging in a strange balancing game between having enough nicotine to stimulate our nicotine receptors, and release dopamine in our brain, and taking so much that we keel over, dead as a dodo. Thankfully the cigarette as a delivery device is not very good at giving us all the nicotine that the tobacco contains – most of the nicotine from the smoke of a cigarette is lost either by us breathing it out again or it being released in between puffs. Depending on your point of view, I suppose you could argue that cigarettes are a good delivery mechanism because they ensure we get enough nicotine to relieve our withdrawals, but not too much that we die. What scientists have realised is that different people have different capacities for dealing with nicotine, depending on how strongly their receptors respond to it. This means that the careful balancing act between getting enough nicotine to give us relief from the withdrawals and having too much that we start to experience the toxic effects is different for different people.

So, there are some people who try a cigarette but simply find it too revolting to continue. While everyone finds their first few cigarettes disgusting, for these people they are truly repellent. This is because they are genetically too sensitive to nicotine to get any enjoyment from it at all, regardless of how much they persevere – for them, the threshold for the toxic effects is too low for them to become smokers. It's thought that their nicotine receptors are simply too sensitive to nicotine. These are the lucky ones – they don't see the appeal in smoking at all. Sometimes, you even hear them say how they really tried to smoke and to like it, but just couldn't.

On the other hand, there are those who have the genes that mean their receptors have just the right affinity for nicotine and that they can also handle large doses of the stuff without experiencing toxic effects. These are your average smoker. Of course, nicotine is still a poison to these people, but their body can handle larger doses than the first group. These people are primed to become addicts. They get the brain rush without the side effects. They don't see how anyone could *not* enjoy smoking. To them, it feels natural because their receptors are perfectly happy.

And the third and final group are the one that my friend's mum falls into. They are genetic freaks (in a nice way). The receptors in their brain are sensitive enough for it to give them some sense of enjoyment, but they are unable to handle it in large doses. This group would never want to be serious, regular smokers, but they can handle the occasional cigarette now and then.

The fact that there are different genetic types when it comes to smoking is very important. The reason for this is that lots of smokers look at the occasional smoker and decide to aim for that, rather than stopping smoking entirely. They think that smoking occasionally will be a nice compromise, and they look at the few people that are able to do this and do not appreciate that they are genetic mutants (again, in a nice way). If they try to aim for this, they will always fail because their genes are against them. It's like me looking at Usain Bolt and thinking, 'Oh, well, I want to run as fast as him, so I will.' It's just not going to happen – Bolt and I have different genes and no amount of hoping will change that. So what these smokers often do is try to cut down and then smoke a few cigarettes a week, which they hate because it's not enough and they feel miserable now, but they stick with it. Then they find something in their life happens – something stressful at work for example – and then they find themselves having a few cigarettes every day. Then something else stressful happens – a row with their partner perhaps – and then, before they know it, they're back to smoking their usual amount and nothing has really changed, except they now associate trying to stop smoking with the pain and discomfort of cutting down and also with failure.

Accept that you will never be one of those people that can have a cigarette once in a while. Let go of that fantasy.

9
Getting to grips with addiction

Smoking is addictive, right? Wrong. Smoking is not, in itself, addictive; it's the nicotine in cigarette smoke that is addictive. This is important to keep in your mind because it's not the act of smoking that you are addicted to, it's simply the chemical that it delivers into your bloodstream. If it were smoking that was addictive, we'd all be happy smoking herbal cigarettes, and we're not.

For the smoker, the thought that they will be without cigarettes is petrifying, but, in reality, the cigarettes are not the problem. It's the nicotine in the cigarette that's the driving force behind the behaviour. As we have just discovered in the last chapter, because of an unfortunate quirk of nature, the cells of our body are covered in receptors that nicotine binds to, and this is why smoking has such an enduring appeal: because it gives us this drug. We are programmed to want nicotine. What's worse, this means that the tobacco industry is using our own bodies against us, for its financial gain. But this isn't the whole story about why people smoke. It's a little bit more complex than just molecules and receptors.

Addiction can be broadly divided into two groups: physiological addiction and psychological addiction. What this means is that addiction can be physical or mental or a combination of both. The power of these two different forms of addiction were very apparent when I worked with drug addicts. Now, before starting this job I knew from medical school that some chemicals, like heroin, are physically very addictive. In a similar way to smoking, there are certain receptors that we have on our cells that opiates (the group of drugs that heroin is in) latch on to. Just as nicotine latches on to nicotine receptors, so opiates latch on to a receptor called, you guessed it, the opiate receptor. And, as happens with nicotine, over time the body starts to make more opiate receptors. When the body has 'up-regulated' the opiate receptors, so the person has to keep taking heroin in order to keep the receptors quiet and stop experiencing withdrawals. And of course the withdrawals from heroin are much, much worse than nicotine. They include shivering, shaking, sweating, goosebumps, explosive diarrhoea, stomach cramps, vomiting, a runny nose, sneezing and insomnia. It's like a very bad bout of flu, so I can understand why people might keep taking heroin, even though they know it's bad for them, in order to avoid these awful withdrawals.

This is why, I thought, people kept using drugs – they were worried about the withdrawals. Doctors have opiate drugs that are similar to heroin and therefore we can replace the heroin with these and then gradually reduce the dose over time. This allows the number of receptors to slowly decrease until, eventually, the number is back to normal and the withdrawals stop (this is the same theory that underpins using nicotine replacement products, like gum and inhalers). I assumed that this physical addiction was all there was to being a drug addict. I was very, very wrong.

What I found astonishing was that actually the physical aspect of heroin addiction is fairly easy to treat by using substitute opiates that are then gradually reduced. In a relatively short period of time, you can get someone off all opiates. But the problem is the psychological aspects of addiction. It is the fact that underlying the physical addiction is something far more powerful – the mind. I learned that it is the psychological aspect of addiction that is the real sticking point for many drug addicts – and, in fact, it is this that makes people struggle to ever get clean or to relapse, regardless of how well they manage their withdrawals. I thought I'd made some miraculous discovery, but actually this is very well known. This is the reason that drug addicts in rehab undergo intense psychotherapy. It's well known that, without changing a heroin addict's psychological dependence on drugs, it's pointless tackling the physical side of things, because they're unlikely to get clean in the first place.

So, with smoking, although nicotine has a physical effect on your cells that results in you experiencing withdrawals – and therefore have an addiction – actually tackling what is going on in your mind when you smoke – how you think about cigarettes – is far more important.

EXERCISE 4: YOUR ONE-DAY SMOKING DIARY

The strange thing about smoking is that the vast majority of times that we smoke, we don't even remember doing it. We go on autopilot. The idea that smoking is an enormous treat is a lie – if it were, we'd remember every cigarette we had, or at least be able to recall them at the end of the day.

In the Introduction I told you that, while you read this book, you were allowed to keep smoking. I now want you to start thinking about smoking when you do it. I'd like you to keep a diary for one day of every time you smoke, with the time and a brief description of what was happening at the time – nothing too elaborate, just a note to yourself to remind yourself of that cigarette.

This is actually quite a boring task, but I make no apologies for how boring it is – this is the whole point. If smoking really gave us something valuable, then it would have a clear, demonstrable improvement on our lives. You'd be able to see this clearly from the diary. You'd at least be able to recall all the cigarettes that you had in a day. We kid ourselves that smoking is something special that gives us something meaningful when, in fact, we spend most of the time doing it without really thinking about it. It's a mindless, meaningless experience. If you don't believe me, try keeping the diary for a few days and see how boring it becomes.

Once you've finished a day of your diary I want you to look back over it and think carefully about the times you were smoking, and if there were any triggers or things that made you feel that you wanted a cigarette. We'll come back to this diary in the next chapter.

10
Cravings

I have two main things to tell you about cravings. The first is that, yes, you will get physical cravings when you stop smoking. You will notice them for the first few days after you stop smoking. In total, they will last for about a month, absolute maximum. For some people it's actually less – only two weeks or so. You should be aware that this is going to happen.

However, the second thing I have to tell you about cravings is that they are the most pathetic, insignificant things you can imagine. The fact that the fear of cravings is what keeps so many people from giving up smoking will seem unimaginable when you have stopped smoking. They have been built up into an enormous thing when, in actual fact, you have been having cravings regularly all the time that you smoked and you hardly even noticed them.

Let me explain. Nicotine, as we have seen, has a natural home on the membranes of the cells in the body. The thing is, though, that it's not very good at staying put. Quite soon after it's latched on, it unlatches itself, floats off and is expelled from the body. So, after you inhale a lungful of smoke, the nicotine level in your blood quickly rises but then quickly dips again. Most of the time the life of a smoker is spent in withdrawal.

The cravings from nicotine are so pathetic that you hardly even notice them. People can sit on a plane for half a day without smoking. They can sit through hours of a play without smoking. As I said before, the cravings are so weak that they don't even wake you up at night. Now compare this to, say, opiate withdrawal, which, as shown in the previous chapter, sees the addict go through a wide range of fairly horrific symptoms – including diarrhoea, stomach cramps, shakes, insomnia and nausea, just to name a few – and you see how mild nicotine withdrawal really is. It's a mild sensation, a slight niggling feeling that typically lasts for about 10–20 seconds. And that's as bad as it gets. For each day you go without smoking, the cravings get less and less. After about a month, they stop.

The key is to remember that, in all of this, there are two things going on – what is actually happening in your body and what is happening in your mind. People can last for hours on end when they accept they can't smoke temporarily – the cravings come and go, hardly registering. In situations when they do not know when they'll be able to smoke, that's when they start panicking. If you tell a smoker that they can smoke again in a few hours' time, for example when they go to the cinema or sit on a train, they'll probably be more or less fine with that. But if you don't tell a smoker how long they have to wait before their next cigarette – if you refuse to give them a time frame – that's likely to be when the cravings will feel unbearable and they won't be able to last an hour without breaking down and pleading with you. So you see, it's not actually the strength of the physical withdrawal that's important here; it's about feeling in control of the withdrawals.

Making a choice to no longer smoke means that you are in control of the withdrawals. Each time you have a withdrawal, they will get less and less, and they will be a reminder that you are ridding your body of this affliction.

Look back at the smoking diary from Exercise 4 in the previous chapter (page 60). Once you've finished your diary, you will see that there were times when you didn't smoke for a while. Actually, from a biological perspective, you were in withdrawal during these periods. Did you notice? Of course not. When you're on the train to work, or in a meeting, you sit there feeling perfectly fine without experiencing withdrawal symptoms.

EXERCISE 5: THE TIME YOU SPEND *NOT* SMOKING

To show you that, actually, you spend most of your time NOT smoking, I want you to calculate the amount of time you spend doing it each day. To do this, multiply the number of cigarettes you usually have by five minutes (the average time it takes to smoke a cigarette). Next work out how long this is in hours, then subtract this number from 24 hours.

If you smoke 20 cigarettes a day, it would be:

- 20 x 5 = 100 minutes
- 100 minutes = 1 hour and 40 minutes

Subtract this from 24 hours and you are left with 22 hours and 20 minutes. That's the vast majority of the day when you don't smoke. In fact, you spend a large proportion of that time in some form of withdrawal, yet it barely even registers.

11

The power of the mind

The brain is the most complex object in the entire universe, and the great news is that each of us has one. The bad news is that with this unbelievably powerful and amazing object, there are no manuals or guides on how to use it. Instead, we all just bumble along doing our best and learning roughly what works and what doesn't work. Given that most of us struggle to work out how to set up a printer on our computer without the aid of several family members, is it any surprise that we struggle sometimes with making the most of our brains? In fact, not only are we not very good at making the most of this incredible, powerful object, but sometimes we accidentally make it do things that we don't want it to do and don't know how to make it stop. We get stuck in traps and dead ends and circles that make no sense. Sometimes we don't realise this has happened and sometimes we do but can't work out how to make it stop. The CBT techniques in this book will help to teach you how to take control of your brain so you can guide it out of the illogical thinking patterns it has got itself into.

I want to tell you a story about how powerful the brain is. In the Second World War there was a man called Henry Beecher. He was an anaesthetist, and he treated the soldiers who had been injured in battle. He was well used to helping people manage with pain from surgery and wounds, and his services were greatly appreciated. When he arrived at war, he found horrific injuries. Many of the soldiers had their legs blown off, shrapnel embedded in their bodies and so on. He knew that these appalling injuries would be agonising and quickly set about preparing morphine. But then he noticed something very strange. Over half of the soldiers reported little or no pain, despite severe wounds, and did not request any pain relief. They were not in shock – they were still able to feel pain; in fact, Beecher noted that they complained about their IV lines just as much as other patients. In peacetime, almost all his patients requested painkillers for injuries of similar severity. This puzzled Beecher as it didn't seem, on a physiological level, to make any sense. Surely the same injury, broadly speaking, should cause the same amount of pain? It was then that he realised he hadn't accounted for one thing: the power of the mind. He realised that for the soldiers, a severe injury was a good thing – it meant that they would be discharged from the army and could return home. For civilians, however, it was a bad thing: a disruption to their life and routine that could mean financial hardship. Beecher realised that it is not necessarily the magnitude of the injury which is important for how a person experiences pain, but the circumstance in which it occurs.

While this is fascinating for those interested in the study of pain, it is also relevant to stopping smoking. What it shows is that our physical experiences are filtered through our mind, and the mind has a tremendous capacity to dictate how we experience things. The mind, essentially, decides how we experience something. Remember this because there will be a time when you question if you are able to stop smoking. You will feel that this is an impossible feat that you will never achieve. Remember Beecher and his soldiers. If they can have their legs blown off and yet their mind can stop it hurting because it appreciates the benefit this injury will have to them, then your mind is more than powerful enough to stop your dependence on nicotine.

In fact, there are many, many stories about the amazing power of the mind. While your mind might have got you into the trap of smoking, it also has the power to get you out of it again. Have faith in the power of your brain. Focus on the positive aspect of stopping smoking – that you know you can do it and you want to achieve this goal, and your brain will make sure it happens.

EXERCISE 6: REASONS TO NOT SMOKE (YOUR 'QUIT LIST')

I want you to go back to the list that you made in Exercise 1 (page 24), where you wrote down all the things that you thought smoking gave you. Now, I want you to write down all the things that NOT smoking would give you. What are the benefits? Why stop smoking? What are your reasons for wanting to no longer smoke? We'll call this your 'quit list'. Even the most die-hard smoker can see some benefits, so list them down, and we'll think about this later in more detail.

12
Willpower

Many people struggle to give up smoking because they believe they lack 'willpower'. They wait around for one day in the future when in some magical way they believe they will suddenly get this mystical 'willpower' from somewhere. This of course is wishful thinking – you may well wake up one day and suddenly decide to stop smoking, but you also might not. It's a big gamble to take, and – given the number of people who smoke throughout their lives, waiting for this to happen – it seems fair to say that it only happens to a small minority of people. It often takes something big and cataclysmic before people suddenly discover this all-elusive willpower – something like being diagnosed with cancer. I have seen so many people who have been given a diagnosis of cancer and then decide to use this to spur them on to stopping. The tragedy is that by then it's too late.

So what can we do about this? Where can we find willpower? The wonderful thing is that you don't need willpower to stop smoking. This sounds like heresy, given that willpower is the one thing that everyone – including stop-smoking counsellors – go on about. It's even on the bottom of adverts for nicotine replacement gums and sprays – 'requires willpower'. But the idea of willpower is based on an entirely unhelpful way of looking at smoking. With willpower there is a delicate balance of short-term gains and long-term gains. For smokers, the short-term benefits of smoking are weighed up against the long-term benefits. Willpower relies on the person being able to mentally tip the balance in favour of the long-term gains and deny themselves the short-term gains. This is difficult to do because, as creatures, human beings tend to focus on short-term benefits. We tend not to be too bothered about the long-term consequences of things if the short-term gains are good. So the smoker who is relying on willpower is relying on their ability to deny themselves something in the here and now for the hope of some benefit in the future. This is why people struggle with willpower because there's always the temptation to give in and allow yourself the short-term gain.

Willpower is also problematic because it allows the smoker to believe that some short-term gains actually exist from smoking, when they do not. Smoking gives you absolutely nothing. In fact, all it does is temporarily alleviate nicotine withdrawal. Nothing more and nothing less. When you understand this, you don't need willpower because there is nothing to outweigh the long-term benefits of not smoking.

13
Life without smoke

For people who have been smoking a long time, especially those who started when they were young, it's often difficult to imagine what life will be like without cigarettes. This feeds into the anxiety about stopping smoking – the unknown and unimaginable is scary and anxiety-provoking. Because of this, the very thought of not smoking scares people. To tackle this anxiety head-on, I want you to play a mind game with yourself. What would it be like if you didn't smoke?

EXERCISE 7: IMAGINE A SMOKE-FREE FUTURE

I want you to get your diary or calendar and pick a date in a few months' time when you have something planned. It can be anything – someone's birthday party or a meal or visiting a friend. Imagine going to that event but that you are a non-smoker. You have absolutely no interest in cigarettes at all.

I want you to go through it in as much detail as you can in your mind. What would you be doing, what would it be like? Every time you come up against a moment when you think, 'I'd light up a cigarette,' allow yourself to pause and remind yourself that in this imaginary world, you are a non-smoker. What are the other non-smokers there doing? They all seem perfectly happy don't they? They're not sitting there miserably wishing they were smokers. What would it feel like? Remember, you don't want a cigarette.

This exercise is purely imaginary. If it makes you feel nervous or anxious, don't worry, you can have a cigarette while you're thinking about this.

Don't do this exercise just once – return to it throughout the day or over a few days. Try it with different future occasions that you have in your diary. Envisage yourself attending these events as a non-smoker. Go through the events in as much detail as your imagination will allow you, really allowing yourself to believe that you don't smoke and don't want a cigarette.

14
Why do people keep smoking?

The simple answer to this is fear. People continue to smoke, despite all the warnings and risks, because they are scared to stop. This is because they fear the prospect of withdrawals. It seems daft to worry about some brief period of discomfort for the long-term benefits, but this is how humans tend to think – we're creatures who dwell in the here and now.

What underlies all of this is something we've already touched upon but is worth reiterating. Smoking sets up a trap in which, once you are hooked, the symptoms that exist when you are NOT smoking are only alleviated by smoking. That's all that smoking gives you – it returns you to the state that non-smokers enjoy all the time. So the smoker is constantly attempting to get back to the same condition they would be in if they didn't smoke in the first place. It's a vicious, cruel and self-perpetuating cycle. The only way to break the cycle is to stop it. Once you've stepped out of the cycle, you'll look back and wonder what on earth you were ever doing in it.

EXERCISE 8: IMAGINE A SMOKE-FREE PAST

This is similar to Exercise 7, but in reverse. I want you to look back a few weeks or months in your diary (depending on how sociable you are) and think back to a recent event you attended when you smoked. Perhaps a dinner party or a night out. Think about when you smoked. The irony is that you probably can't remember many of the cigarettes you actually smoked because, as we mentioned earlier, most cigarettes aren't particularly enjoyable – they're simply functional in that they get nicotine into your system. But try to think about what happened on this day and the times you smoked and how it made you feel.

Now I want to take this thought experiment one step further. If you'd stopped smoking on that day, you would be a non-smoker. You'd be sitting here, reading this, no longer hooked to cigarettes, entirely free. So I now want you to think back to that date in the past that you picked and imagine that you stopped smoking then. Sit and think about today and what that would feel like. You've stopped smoking already so you have no withdrawals and no anxiety associated with not smoking. You are just free from cigarettes. What does that feel like?

Don't worry if this imagination game doesn't come easily to you at first – practise thinking about the day in the past and what it would feel like to be a non-smoker. Remember, you're not longing for a cigarette because you're a non-smoker. What I want you to think about is what it must feel like to be a non-smoker and to realise that if you *had* decided to stop on that date, you'd now be entirely free, and to imagine how that would make you feel.

PART THREE

YOUR THOUGHTS ABOUT SMOKING

I've already mentioned that the most difficult part to quitting is not coping with the physical symptoms but changing the way you think about smoking. In this section we are going to look at some of the thinking that underpins people's feelings about smoking. We will examine some of the ideas, thoughts and feelings that keep us tied to our relationship with cigarettes, and how these may be holding you back.

15
The lies we tell ourselves

Although the mind is incredibly powerful, where smoking is concerned it has fallen into a trap. To free ourselves from this trap, we first have to understand it. Before you read any further, I want you to get out the notes you made for Exercise 1 (page 24), and look at them again. Everything that you wrote down in Exercise 1 is an illusion. These 'reasons you smoke' might seem very real, but they are not. Instead, everything on this list is your mind's attempt to justify something that doesn't make sense.

Deep down, we all know that smoking is bad for us. It costs an incredible amount of money and, ultimately, it's likely to either kill or disable us. It is the source of immeasurable suffering to both us and those around us. In the mind, this sets up a bit of a quandary. We want to do it because if we don't we experience withdrawals, but we know it is bad for us and should not do it. In psychology, this problem is called 'cognitive dissonance' – when our thoughts are in conflict with one another and this contradiction results in us feeling uncomfortable with our thoughts. Part of becoming a smoker

79

is that your mind finds ways to resolve this 'dissonance' so that you can continue smoking without experiencing the mental conflict. It does this by coming up with 'cognitive distortions' – arguments that, on the face of it, might seem logical and that allow you to keep smoking. Part of the path to becoming a non-smoker again is picking apart these arguments that your mind relies on to justify you smoking.

If I ask you to rationalise why you smoke, you'll probably come back with a whole list of reasons. Every single one of them will be based on false logic. They are tricks of the mind that have been created in order to avoid the discomfort you would experience if you acknowledged that what you do makes no sense.

Below are some of the common justifications that are really cognitive distortions. I will show you how each of these thinking patterns is illogical and flawed. Now, you might find some of these rationalisations difficult to read. That's okay. They're hard to read because they are challenging the justifications you have set up in your mind to explain why you smoke. If you do find them difficult, take a break and come back to them. Try to keep an open mind. Allow yourself time to think about them. They make sense don't they? The reason your mind tries to find ways not to accept these rationalisations is because they challenge the illogical thinking patterns that enable you to keep smoking. Remember, smoking gives you nothing. Stopping smoking does not remove anything meaningful or important.

'SMOKING HELPS ME WHEN I'M FEELING STRESSED'

Smoking itself does nothing to stop you feeling stressed. If anything, it actually makes you more stressed because you have to keep doing it to avoid withdrawals. The sense of relief you get from smoking is a direct result of the fact that you smoke. Let me explain this, because it's key to understanding the smoking trap that your mind plays on you. When we smoke we set up an unwinnable game with our bodies. As we've seen in Chapter 10, nicotine is not very good at staying in the body for any appreciable time, so smokers spend most of their days in a constant state of mild withdrawal. This low-level discomfort that we experience periodically is only relieved by smoking, which of course then means that shortly afterwards we will be in withdrawal again, and the sorry cycle continues. The situation is accompanied by the small niggling feeling that at some point we will need to address the withdrawals and smoke a cigarette – so, when we do, we feel that this has helped us with our stress levels. There is nothing inherent in a cigarette that calms us. In fact, smoking raises blood pressure and heart rate, so, if anything, it contributes to stress.

'SMOKING HELPS ALLEVIATE BOREDOM'

Smoking is something to do. That's what smokers tell themselves. But actually, is there anything more boring than smoking? Smoking does not mentally stimulate you – it's a dull, repetitious activity. Are non-smokers more bored than smokers? Do non-smokers sit there staring into the middle distance, wishing they were smoking because they are so mind-numbingly bored? Of course not. Look at the diary you wrote in Exercise 4 (page 60). At no point after any of the cigarettes you had did you return to whatever you were doing and say to someone, 'Wow, I've just been smoking. God, that was interesting.' It's dull. There is absolutely nothing mentally stimulating about putting dried, rolled-up foliage into your mouth and lighting it.

Smoking provides a way of punctuating your time – something to break the monotony of your day. But then so do lots of activities. Going to the toilet does the same, but you don't do that 20 times a day just as a way of alleviating boredom, do you? Smoking is not really about boredom, it's about getting nicotine into your system. We tell ourselves that it's about boredom because this is a way of justifying it to ourselves. There is nothing interesting about cigarettes. They do not stimulate our minds in any way. If you need something to do to punctuate your day, you can make a cup of tea, get up and walk around, or go and get some fresh air. This is what non-smokers do and they are not more bored than smokers. Feel reassured by this – it's just more evidence that, while it sometimes feels like it, smoking does not really give you anything.

'IT HELPS ME CONCENTRATE'

I used to justify smoking by telling myself that it helped me concentrate. This was the perfect lie to tell myself because in my job I need to concentrate. But I knew, even as I said this to myself, that it didn't make any sense. The times I really needed to concentrate – when I was seeing a patient, for example, or doing a complicated procedure – I couldn't smoke. I managed to do these tasks perfectly well without a cigarette. Ah, I said to myself, but when I write it helps me concentrate. But actually, the more I thought about this, the more I knew it wasn't true. If anything, cigarettes interrupted my train of thought because I'd have to stop typing, light up, sit back and smoke one. When I then got back to writing, it would often take a minute or two to remind myself of what I'd been typing and to pick up my train of thought again. Not only did it not help me concentrate, it actually hindered my concentration.

Remember, non-smokers are not plagued by poor concentration. The reason having a cigarette gives the illusion of helping with concentration is because without smoking you are in withdrawal and this distracts you. But it's smoking that caused these withdrawals! So, actually, being a smoker decreases your ability to concentrate because you are regularly experiencing tiny withdrawals, and this takes over your mind and affects your ability to concentrate. When you have a cigarette, you then temporarily relieve this withdrawal and return to the same level of ability to concentrate as non-smokers enjoy the whole time. However, you experience this as it helping you concentrate. In fact, all smoking has done is temporarily help you stop being distracted. There is nothing inherent within a cigarette that helps people concentrate. If you gave a cigarette to a non-smoker, they wouldn't suddenly experience a surge in their ability to concentrate. So if you stop smoking then, after the initial withdrawals, you will return to the same ability to concentrate that all non-smokers enjoy.

'SMOKING HELPS ME RELAX'

This is an illusion and you can clearly show this by doing a simple test on yourself. Next time you have a cigarette, check the effect it has on your heart. You can work out your heart rate – the number of times your heart beats in a minute – by taking your pulse for 30 seconds and then doubling that number. Take your heart rate while at rest before having a cigarette and then repeat this afterwards. What's happened? Your heart rate will have shot up. I did this on myself before stopping smoking and was horrified to see that I had a resting pulse of about 60 but when I smoked it shot up to over 100. Now, a heart rate of over 100 is similar to what you'd expect after going for a run – hardly very physically relaxing.

Again, as with all the other tricks your mind has played on you, smoking gives you the *illusion* of relaxing. When you are not smoking, you are depending on the last cigarette you had and then on edge waiting for your next one. So smoking does not relax you; instead it's smoking that causes the agitation, which is alleviated by another cigarette. Massages help you relax. Stroking a puppy helps you relax. Smoking does not.

'I ENJOY SMOKING'

Do you? What do you actually enjoy about it? The smell? Being a slave to something that you know is going to kill you? The expense? I enjoy all sorts of things – going to the theatre, reading books, swimming. But I don't have to do these things repeatedly throughout the day in order to simply feel satisfied. The reason people think that they enjoy cigarettes is because of the temporary sense of relief they provide from the niggling withdrawals of nicotine. That's not really enjoying something. It's like repeatedly ducking your head under water so you can enjoy the sensation of not drowning when you temporarily stop.

'I'VE GOT TO DIE OF SOMETHING'

I used to say this to myself all the time. I liked saying it because it sounded flippant and slightly edgy. It sounded even better coming from a doctor because people would be temporarily silenced as they thought, 'Well, yes, I suppose he's right.' I knew deep within that this was daft logic, but, still, it's the sort of thing that *sounds* like a credible argument. It is, of course, absolute rubbish. Firstly, unless you are suicidal, people don't want to die. Doing something that knowingly increases your chance of an early death is plain daft. You have to die of something, but you don't have to do it 20 years sooner.

Also, there is a fundamental flaw to this argument because smoking might not kill you – it might incapacitate you instead. Some of the diseases that smoking gives you are, arguably, far worse than death. The idea of lying in a bed, immobile and unable to do anything for yourself is a lot of people's idea of hell, and yet this is what you're gambling with when you smoke, as it significantly increases the risk of strokes. I also don't want my legs to need amputating or to go blind, but again, this is what smoking can cause. There is also the risk of developing chronic obstructive pulmonary disease

– COPD – which leaves the sufferer constantly unable to get their breath. Pretty much everyone with COPD has smoked. I saw lots of these people in hospital, and it was so horrifying watching them desperately gasping for each breath non-stop through the day and night; I sometimes couldn't bring myself to look at them. Smoking also increases the risk of small strokes that damage the brain and can change the blood flow to the brain, resulting in dementia. Recent research has shown that smokers are at nearly 50 per cent increased risk of developing dementia compared to non-smokers. You've got to die of something, but no one wants to be horribly incapacitated for years beforehand.

'IF I STOP SMOKING I'LL GAIN WEIGHT'

Are people that don't smoke fatter than smokers? No. The irony is that people who don't smoke look younger, don't smell and are fitter. But there is a myth that people who smoke are slimmer – probably perpetuated by the images of young, attractive, skinny models smoking who say they do so because it suppresses appetite. Lots of people – particularly women – justify not stopping smoking because they are afraid that they will suddenly put on weight. We'll look at this issue again in more detail towards the end of this part of the book, but let's touch upon it now too.

The main reason that some people put on weight after they stop smoking is because they have not properly resolved in their minds that smoking actually gives them nothing. It does absolutely zilch for them but they continue to believe that they are missing out on something. To fill this imaginary void, they eat. People who stop smoking put on weight because they start to eat more. They do this because they want to comfort themselves as they believe that they are denying themselves something – cigarettes – so they compensate with something else – food. But if you accept that the act of smoking is an empty experience, giving you nothing real or meaningful, then there is no reason to substitute this with food. Of course, this may sound easier said than done to you at the moment, but there are some simple ways to make sure that you keep yourself in check and don't put on weight when you stop, which we'll cover in Chapter 26. When you've gone through the process of stopping using this technique, your mind will no longer view stopping smoking as giving anything up, so you won't feel the need to substitute it with anything. This comes naturally out of the process, so please don't worry about it.

'I LIKE THE TASTE'

Think back to when you had your first cigarette. No one thinks, 'Oh, that's a nice taste,' when they inhale their cigarette. The 'taste' of a cigarette is a marketing myth pushed by cigarette manufacturers to try to differentiate themselves in a marketplace where there's actually nothing intrinsically appealing about their product. 'Smoother taste' just means it's less harsh than usual cigarettes. Smokers actually taste disgusting – ask any non-smoker who has kissed a smoker. The only reason smokers don't realise this is because we've killed off so many of our taste buds (don't worry, they grow back when you stop smoking) so that we don't notice it.

So, to conclude, all of the benefits you think you get from smoking are actually tricks of the mind. All the benefits you *think* you get are simply the temporary relief of the withdrawals that you are experiencing. We convince ourselves that cigarettes give us a benefit but, in reality, all they do is return us to the state that non-smokers enjoy all the time. Every cigarette you smoke perpetuates the addiction and therefore sets up the need for the next one. The only way to step out of this vicious cycle is to stop smoking.

16
Thinking errors

We've just seen how the mind plays tricks on us to justify some of our behaviours. Such 'thinking errors' tend to follow set patterns. These patterns undermine our ability to see a problem clearly and result in us feeling overwhelmed. This is the case for all sorts of things, such as depression and anxiety, but it also underpins some of the thinking errors seen in smokers. With smoking, these thought patterns stop us from feeling in control and able to change our behaviour. This is particularly true if we've tried to stop smoking before and failed.

Below is a list of some of the common thinking errors that smokers make when they think about stopping.

OVERGENERALISATION

This is when we take one negative event as evidence of an underlying pattern. For example, with smoking: 'I tried to give up smoking once and I failed. Therefore I'll always fail and it's pointless trying again.' Or: 'My friend/relative found it difficult to stop smoking, therefore I will.'

ALL-OR-NOTHING THINKING

This is when we see things as being black or white, rather than accepting that there are shades in between. So, for smoking, all-or-nothing thinking would include thoughts such as: 'I can't cope with stress or difficulties, so there's no way I'll be able to stop smoking.' Or: 'If I can't smoke at a party, I won't enjoy myself.'

MENTAL FILTER

This is when we fixate on a single negative detail and ignore the positive: 'I can't bear the idea of withdrawals, so stopping smoking is going to be horrendous.'

DISCOUNTING THE POSITIVE

This is when we maintain negative beliefs about ourselves and our abilities by ignoring the positive achievements or experiences in our lives. With smoking, this might include thoughts such as: 'I never achieve anything, so why should I be able to achieve this?'

EMOTIONAL REASONING

This is when we make assumptions about things based purely on emotions. For example: 'I feel scared about stopping smoking, so therefore I'm not going to succeed.' Or: 'The thought of stopping smoking makes me feel stressed, so I'm going to fail.'

JUMPING TO CONCLUSIONS

This is when we draw negative conclusions without having all the facts to support them. In the case of smoking, this often takes the form of 'predicting the future' – whereby we predict we are going to fail before we've even tried, and so don't see the point in trying.

EXERCISE 9: YOUR OWN THINKING ERRORS

It's important that you recognise the thinking errors that you are making about smoking. In order to do this, I want you to go back to the event in the future that you imagined in Exercise 7 (page 71). Using this event, do the following:

Think about the future situation and write down what it is. Now, close your eyes and imagine yourself again there as vividly as you can. Write down any negative thoughts you have when you imagine not smoking in this situation. Be honest with yourself about the anxieties and worries. Finally, think carefully and critically about these feelings. Use the list above to understand the thinking errors that are going on, and write them down.

You can repeat this for as many other situations related to smoking as you want. The more you do it, the more thinking errors you'll uncover and be able to recognise.

Here's an example:

Situation: At the pub

Negative thoughts: I'm weak and will want a cigarette. My friends will laugh at me if they discover that I've tried to stop and won't support me. I'll have a miserable time because I won't be able to smoke. I'll feel isolated and alone if I don't smoke.

Thinking errors: All-or-nothing thinking, overgeneralisation and jumping to conclusions.

Now you try it:

Situation:

Negative thoughts:

Thinking errors:

Next, take a look at your list and think of alternative responses to the situations that do not involve a thinking error. Don't worry if this takes a bit of time or you find it tricky at first. It sometimes helps if you imagine that a friend or relative has come to you with this problem and wants your help. What would you say to someone to help *them* think differently and in a more positive way about a situation?

So, with the example of the pub, you might respond:

'We all have times when we feel weak, but there is no reason for you to think that you are any weaker than other people. Some of your friends might laugh at you, but you don't know for sure that they will and, besides, others will be supportive. What you are doing is an incredible achievement. You won't be isolated, lots of other people don't smoke, and they do not feel alone when they go out.'

17

Reasons to continue vs reasons to quit

Now I want to go back to the list that you made in Exercise 3, your list of 'reasons to continue smoking' (page 47). I guarantee, without ever seeing your list, that it will be identical (give or take a few items) to that of every person who has ever smoked. The reason for this is not that these are real reasons to continue smoking but that the mind tends to follow the same, predictable patterns in the way it makes errors of thinking. There are only so many ways of arguing that black is white, and similarly there are only so many ways of convincing yourself that doing something bad and meaningless is actually good and worthwhile.

So take a look at that list and allow yourself to think about it critically. To do this best, you need to be able to detach yourself personally from smoking and your own personal feelings about it. You need to try to be objective about this whole thing, and so, to help you do this, I want you to put smoking 'on trial' in the next exercise. Some people like to do this by writing it down, but personally I think it's quite effective if you actually wait until everyone is out of the house and do it by yourself in front of the mirror.

EXERCISE 10: SMOKING ON TRIAL

I want you to imagine that you are a lawyer in a legal case. The stakes here are high – someone's life is on the line (yours). First of all, put the case forward for continuing smoking. You already have the information for this from Exercises 1 and 3. Imagine putting forward this argument in front of a judge and jury, and be as persuasive as you can be. Use emotive phrases; play on their emotions. Cigarettes are on trial and you are defending them.

Now, I want you to switch sides and imagine that you are the prosecution barrister in this case. Put forward the argument *against* smoking. Start by explaining the benefits of no longer smoking, as you outlined in your 'quit list' in Exercise 6 (page 68). In true Perry Mason style I want you to demolish the opposition, by blowing the case supporting smoking out of the water. Use the things you learned in the last two sections about the way the mind plays tricks on us and the errors that develop in our thinking to challenge each of the points that you put forward in defence of cigarettes. You need to convince the judge and jury that the arguments in support of continuing to smoke are a load of nonsense.

The cases you make in Exercise 10 reflect what goes on inside your head when you smoke. There is part of you that is screaming for you to stop; it is scared of what you are doing to yourself and hates being a slave to nicotine. But there is the other part of your brain that tries to convince you that everything is okay, and that you shouldn't worry; it does this by generating myths, illusions and distortions in order to justify carrying on this behaviour.

If you were sitting on that jury, whom would you believe? Of course, the case against smoking is far stronger than the case for it – in fact, if you've been a good lawyer, you'll have shown that there isn't even a case. The arguments in favour of continuing to smoke are all lies, fallacies, misunderstandings, illusions and distortions. The defence has no case; the prosecution has clearly won.

18
The stages of change

Fundamental to stopping smoking is change. It is what stopping smoking is all about: you currently do something and you are going to change your behaviour. How people change and the psychological process that occurs is of great interest to doctors and therapists. In the 1980s a model of behaviour change was drawn up that is still relevant today. It describes the psychological stages that people go through when they are considering changing a behaviour. This model can be applied to all sorts of behaviours, not just smoking, and there's a lot of medical literature written about it. It's kind of a big deal, especially in things like drug addiction. And, of course, as we've seen, even though smoking can sometimes feel as though it has some mystical, strange hold over you, it is actually simply a drug addiction.

So, the model of behaviour change is relevant here because it helps set out the psychological process that people go through when they start the journey towards quitting smoking. You can work out where in the model you are and where you'd like to be. People tend to move from one stage to the other, but sometimes get stuck at a stage. Alternatively, sometimes smokers take a step back – usually from stage 3 to 2.

Here are the five stages to change:

1

Pre-contemplation: The person has no intention of stopping smoking and resists any attempts to change this. They show all the cognitive distortions discussed in Chapter 15 and refuse to consider that any of these might be untrue.

2

Contemplation: The person recognises that smoking is a problem for them and wishes that they could stop. They have begun to understand that some of the justifications that they tell themselves about why they continue smoking don't entirely make sense and might be based on false logic. They want to stop but are too scared. They often feel tormented and frustrated. Most adult smokers are at this stage, and the thing to remember is it's easy to move to the next stage.

3

Preparation: The smoker is actively making steps to stop smoking and has a plan to do this. They begin to develop solutions to problems they predict they might encounter.

4

Action: The person has now stopped smoking and is a non-smoker again. In order to do this they have made changes to their behaviours, their understanding of themselves and how they define themselves in relation to cigarettes.

5

Maintenance: The person is working to prevent relapse and to build on the action phase (4). This phase usually starts after about three months of stopping smoking, when the novelty of having stopped has worn off and the initial elation of being free of cigarettes has passed.

Don't worry if you look at this list and think you're at stage 1 or 2. This doesn't mean you can't shift where you are, and, indeed, there's very good evidence that even people at stage 1 can be catapulted into action when their thinking is gently challenged using CBT methods. This is because the reasons that people use to justify smoking to themselves are very weak and easily destroyed – as we have seen in the Chapter 15. Being based on false logic, they are defenceless against the logic of reason. That's not to say that you might not find it challenging or anxiety-provoking, initially at least, but if you relax and allow yourself to think about the arguments for and against smoking, you will realise that the excuses you make around why you smoke are embarrassingly illogical.

If you're at stage 1, then you've already made a massive step forward without even realising it by picking up this book and reading this far. There is a part of you that *does* want to stop. Keep going and continue to do the exercises, and this part will continue to grow.

Whatever stage you're at, don't panic yourself by looking forward and thinking about stopping smoking – or maintaining this once you've taken action. Take small steps and simply keep reading and doing the exercises. Moving through the stages is a process that happens naturally through gently challenging your thinking.

19
Getting stuck

The reasons you might get stuck at one of the stages of change, or slip back a stage, follow a fairly predictable pattern: the logical thinking starts to gets crowded out again by illogical arguments that favour smoking. So, let's spend some time reminding ourselves of the reasons people give to themselves about why they should stay at stages 1, 2 or 3 and not progress to stages 4 and 5. Some of these arguments have been touched on before, but it's important to emphasise them because they form the basis of the smoking trap into which people get stuck. These are the bricks and mortar of the cell in which every smoker has been incarcerated. The good news is, the walls of that prison cell are easily demolished. Take another look at the list you made in Exercise 3 (page 47), your list of 'reasons to continue smoking', then read through the following excuses:

'IT'S NOT THE RIGHT TIME'

I've got some news for you: it's never the right time to stop smoking. Or, depending on how you look at it, it's always the right time. The fact is that there will always be something going on in your life: something that's stressful or difficult or there to preoccupy you. The number one thing I hear time and time again is the phrase: 'I will stop, just not now.' If not now, when? To show you what I mean, take your diary and look at it. Pick a random month and look at all the things you did over that time period. Undoubtedly, there will be some things that were stressful. That's because life is full of stressful or preoccupying events. We'll look at how exactly to plan to stop smoking and pick the day that's right for you to quit later, but, rest assured, the 'one day' argument is the oldest cop-out in the book. What will it take for that 'one day' to come? When you get cancer? When a doctor tells you they'll have to remove your leg? When you go blind?

'I NEED IT TO CONCENTRATE'

Smoking does not help you concentrate. There have been many studies looking at the ability of nicotine to enhance performance and there is not a shred of evidence that it improves concentration or ability to perform tasks one jot. Remember, the only thing that smoking does is temporarily relieve the mild niggling sensation of withdrawal that all smokers experience. Smoking a cigarette temporarily returns you to the state that all non-smokers enjoy all the time. Non-smokers do not concentrate less than smokers. In fact, they concentrate better because they are not being distracted by the low-level niggle of withdrawal symptoms. Stopping smoking will actually help you concentrate more.

If you need a break from what you're doing, then get up, walk around, make a cup of tea – this is what everyone who doesn't smoke does. This is what is normal. Remember, you can concentrate in the theatre or cinema, and you don't smoke there. You can concentrate and focus on an aeroplane or train – people happily read books or listen to music, for example. Smoking only gives the illusion of being able to help you concentrate because it stops you from being distracted by the desire to smoke.

I had totally convinced myself that I could only write when I was smoking. I was absolutely petrified that when I stopped, I'd be unable to write. And do you know what happened when I stopped smoking? Writing was actually easier. Why? Because I wasn't lighting up a cigarette every five minutes, dropping the ash on the keyboard, sitting back and daydreaming while I puffed away. The irony was that the signs had been there all along: I remember noticing that when I was really on a roll with writing and the words were flowing and I was engrossed in the article I was writing, the cigarette would often go untouched in the ashtray and burn right down to the butt before I realised that I hadn't actually smoked it. I'd then light another one, I'd be distracted and then my train of thought would be broken.

At work, where I wasn't allowed to smoke in my office, I actually became more productive. Why? Because I wasn't going out for a cigarette every so often and disrupting my flow of work. I wasn't sitting rushing through one task so I could pop out and smoke before starting something new. Smoking not only didn't help me concentrate, it was actually doing the opposite. However, it gave me the *illusion* of helping me concentrate because it temporarily stopped me thinking about cigarettes by alleviating the niggling withdrawals.

'IT MAKES ME HAPPY'

This is an interesting one. Research has shown that smokers *think* that smoking boosts their mood, but, in actual fact, in studies looking at this, it's been shown that this is entirely false. Smoking only gives the *illusion* of improving your mood because it temporarily alleviates the withdrawal symptoms you experience. This is an awful, tragic situation to be in and is true for all smokers. It means that smokers spend the majority of their day slightly unhappy because they're not smoking, only for them to be returned to the normal level of happiness that non-smokers enjoy all the time for a brief moment when they smoke. It's like playing thumping, headache-inducing music all day so that, periodically, you can turn it off and enjoy the quietness.

'I'LL MISS IT TOO MUCH'

In Chapter 2 I talked about smoking as being a relationship with cigarettes and said that I wanted you to view it in these terms. Most people have had, at some point in their lives, a relationship that in hindsight was not quite as perfect as you thought at the time. Remember, your relationship with cigarettes is the most damaging, toxic relationship you have ever had. It will take everything from you. It is like dating a homicidal maniac who's out to kill you. Cigarettes, by no small stretch of the imagination, are not a 'keeper'. You will not miss something that gives you absolutely nothing. It's like missing air pollution or herpes. There are no real benefits from being in this relationship with cigarettes, and instead, only negatives. The benefits you think exist are just illusions, distortions and myths.

'IT HELPS ME COPE'

People who do not smoke have just as many things going on in their lives as people who do smoke. How do you think they cope? The fact is that they cope in exactly the same way that you cope. What do I mean? Smoking doesn't really help you cope with anything in life. It doesn't make things change in the outside world any more than hopping on one foot does. It gives you the illusion that it helps you cope simply because it deals with one additional difficulty that the non-smoker doesn't have: it temporarily alleviates that niggling feeling of nicotine withdrawal. That's not helping you cope! That's simply providing you with an additional stress that you have to cope with – and then taking the credit for alleviating all the stress, when actually all it's done is momentarily reduce the stress that it caused in the first place: the nicotine withdrawal.

'IT'S WHO I AM'

Out of every excuse, this is the one I most identified with. I allowed smoking to define me, and the thought of stopping horrified me because I didn't know who I'd be if I didn't smoke. I look back at myself and feel intense sorrow for the person I was – that I allowed one simple, daft behaviour to define who I was. I eat a banana every day for breakfast, but I don't define myself by that.

Again, this was just another justification for not stopping – a rather pathetic attempt to convince myself that smoking was important to me in a deep and personal way. I've actually sat in front of quite a few heroin and crack addicts who have said exactly the same thing to me about stopping using drugs: that they were scared because it was who they were. The first time I heard someone say this, I thought how tragic it was – who, in their right mind, would want to be a heroin addict, let alone feel that it defined them? But it's exactly the same thing as being a smoker. Smoking is not an achievement or label to define yourself by.

You spend the majority of your day not smoking. Don't define yourself by it. Don't allow yourself to be defined by your addiction. You are more than a smoker, and this will continue when you're a non-smoker.

'I'VE TRIED BEFORE AND FAILED'

There is nothing more disheartening than having tried incredibly hard to stop smoking, only to find yourself relapse. I completely understand the frustration and annoyance that those in this position feel. It's incredibly tough to be facing doing the same thing again, knowing that you might fail. But, for a moment, allow yourself to step back from your own situation and think about this objectively. If someone came to you who had tried to stop smoking but failed, what would you say to them? Would you say: 'Oh, don't worry then, just keep doing it and don't bother trying again'? Of course you wouldn't. Failing is not a reason to stop attempting something; it's a reason to try again.

Some smokers have to try to quit a dozen times before they succeed, but the thing to remember is that the vast majority of smokers who try to quit succeed eventually. Sometimes these things take a bit of time and trial and error. Remember, you're trying to reprogramme the most complex object in the universe. Sometimes you don't get it quite right and need to do it again. Stop thinking about this as a failure and think of it more as a setback. Think carefully about what caused you to slip up last time and focus on this; think of a strategy to avoid this the next time you try. Please, don't give up on yourself. You deserve better than that.

In fact, there's good evidence to show that having previously tried to give up is associated with eventual success. It's not clear the exact reason for this, but it's thought that smokers learn from past attempts and apply this knowledge to the next attempt. Sometimes it takes several goes, but each time you learn something new about your relationship with cigarettes and why you slipped up the last time. It's a bit like negotiating your way through a maze. Some people might get out in the first attempt, but others have to take a few wrong turnings first. With each wrong turning, you learn that it was a dead end, so you make sure you don't take that turning when you try again.

'I'LL LOSE MY FRIENDS'

We'll deal with social situations a bit later in the book, but, suffice to say, smoking is actually one of the most antisocial activities that someone can do. You may well have a number of friends you smoke with, but – as more and more people quit – smokers will become more and more isolated. It is a dwindling social circle and is only getting smaller. You are putting out deckchairs on the *Titanic*.

If your friends are *only* there because you smoke with them, then they are not really friends. They're just smoking buddies. It's sometimes hard to appreciate this, but if your relationship can't withstand you no longer smoking, then that relationship wasn't worth having in the first place. You have real friends and it's the relationships with these people that will endure, regardless of whether you smoke or not.

Once you come to understand that smoking gives you nothing, the desire to do it will vanish in a, well, puff of smoke. This means you can still hang out with smokers if you want. You can still go outside with a friend after a meal to keep him or her company if they want to smoke. You don't smoke with them because you know that you get nothing from it and it does nothing for you. All you have done is climb out of the trap that your smoking friends are still stuck in.

20
Heroin

Over the course of my career, I've sat in front of a lot of heroin addicts and talked to them about what they do and why they do it. I've heard every excuse and every reason for them to continue being addicts – why they are scared of stopping heroin and countless reasons and arguments as to why they need it and why they can't stop. Smoking is no different because, just like heroin, it's simply a drug addiction, and there are clear parallels between smokers and heroin addicts in the psychological mechanisms they use to justify their behaviour.

I don't want you to be scared by the heroin comparison – of course, there are many differences, not least that smoking is legal. However, it's useful because all the same excuses and same justifications are used by heroin addicts as by smokers. Also, the same psychological techniques that are used to challenge heroin addicts about their addiction and get them to move towards abstinence are the same for smokers.

The other reason the comparison is useful is that most people can see the absurdity of heroin addiction. It's considered one of the world's great evils. To the average person, it makes no sense and is actually quite horrifying. The thought of injecting (or smoking) a highly addictive substance like heroin, that the body doesn't need in any way, that is dangerous and potentially lethal, that is financially costly and that takes away people's control over their lives, is awful. Yet how is this different from smoking? It's not. Let yourself imagine you are sitting in front of a heroin addict and they are trying to justify their addiction to you – all the excuses about it helping them cope, making them relax and so on. Imagine all the counterarguments you would give them. It's exactly the same for smoking.

The really shocking thing is that smoking is actually worse than heroin from a physical health perspective – a smoker is statistically more likely to die from smoking than a heroin addict is from taking heroin. It is actually more risky to your health than heroin. Now of course I'm not saying that you should switch smoking cigarettes to smoking heroin! The point of this isn't to scare you or upset you, but it's interesting to see how, when it's someone else's addiction that we are looking at objectively, we can easily spot how their justifications for their actions don't make any sense and don't stand up to logical reasoning. It shouldn't be so hard to put up a mirror to ourselves and realise that the smoker is not that different to the heroin addict.

21
Ambivalence

The real reason that people keep smoking is that they are scared. Deep down, this is the real reason you smoke. The sad thing about this is that, really, the only thing to be scared about is continuing to smoke, not stopping. But, as we have seen, the brain doesn't always work in a logical way. The fear of a few weeks of withdrawals – even though, smokers spend most of their lives in some degree of withdrawal – is greater than the fear of dying or being disabled. This is what is going on deep inside in your mind, and this fear is keeping you smoking.

Rather than focus on the negative effects of continuing to smoke, it's often helpful to focus on the positive benefits of quitting. If you're feeling stuck and struggling to move forward through the stages of change outlined in Chapter 18, then don't panic. Try this simple exercise to help refocus your mind on what you want to achieve.

EXERCISE 11: THE GOLDEN THREE

Go back to the list you created in Exercise 6, your 'quit list' (page 68). Most people will have a combination of health and social reasons on this list. I want you to rank your top three reasons. These are the 'golden three' of the list – the three main reasons, above all else, that are your motivation for stopping. Now, write them on a piece of card and carry this card with you in your wallet or purse. Every so often, take this card out and read it to yourself. Then close your eyes and imagine those things becoming a reality for you. How would you feel? Allow yourself to have that feeling for a few moments. These three things are going to become a motivational mantra for you. So, if one of the things in your golden three is the cost of smoking, then say to yourself: 'Every day that I don't smoke, I'm saving more and more money.' Or, if it's health, say to yourself: 'Every day that I don't smoke, my body is becoming healthier and healthier.'

22
Desire

Another obstacle to stopping is that smokers often think that they can't stop until they no longer *want* to smoke. They assume that to move from stage 3 (preparation) to 4 (action) in the stages of change (see Chapter 18), they have to have absolutely no desire to smoke. This isn't true. It's unlikely that you'll experience some magical moment when you will feel you simply don't want to light up, because you are addicted to nicotine. What's happening here is that you are confusing desire (wanting to do something) with addiction. To put it another way, it feels like you *want* to smoke, but this is not really desire, it's addiction. This is an important point to realise because it's the addiction that's making you smoke, not a love of smoking.

Waiting for some improbable point when you simply have no interest in smoking is another trick of the mind to put you off having to take action. Lots of smokers will experience some ambivalence around stopping smoking right up until the moment they do it. It's fine to feel like this. What we're trying to do is allow the part of the brain that wants to stop to feel stronger and more confident – so the mind can listen to this voice rather than the one telling it to continue.

It's sometimes helpful to think of it as two voices sitting on each shoulder – a devil and an angel, if you want. The devil will keep whispering in your ear its reasons to keep smoking. It will use every trick in the book to introduce uncertainty and confusion. Everything it whispers in your ear is based on false logic and illusions. It's a powerful voice though. On the other shoulder is the angel. This is the voice that is providing all the logical reasons why you should stop smoking. Don't wait for the devil on the shoulder to disappear entirely – simply start listening to the angel on the other shoulder more, and the devil's voice will lose its power and eventually waste away.

Remind yourself that the part of your brain that is coming up with the justifications for smoking – the devil on your shoulder – is just scared. It's panicking because it knows that all its arguments disintegrate the minute any logic is applied, so it's making a last-ditch attempt to keep you smoking by suggesting that you have to wait until you never want to smoke again. As a smoker, you are addicted to nicotine, so while you continue to smoke that addiction will remain – and the illogical part of your brain can always use this to justify continuing smoking. Don't listen to it. Remember that while you might experience a physical craving, this is mild and soon passes; it is not a reason to allow your brain to convince you to continue smoking.

23
Coping strategies

As we've seen, smoking gives the *illusion* of helping you cope with things in your everyday life. It doesn't really do this, but the belief is strong, so it's worth spending some time on this aspect of smoking.

Smoking itself represents what psychologists call a 'maladaptive coping strategy'. This means that it's a behaviour that someone has developed that appears to help them, but actually doesn't. The problem with smoking is that it's 'over-practised' – that is, smokers do it so often throughout the day, that it becomes habitual. Habitual behaviour can, in itself, be comforting. This doesn't mean that smoking in itself is comforting, but it does mean that the familiar *act* of smoking can be comforting and so feel as though it's helping you cope with whatever stress or difficulty you are facing. This is because smokers have got stuck in a rut whereby they mistakenly think that, because they do it so often during the day, the repetitious nature of lighting up a cigarette is helping them.

How exactly does smoking seem to do this? Well, it works on two levels. The first is that when we do something a lot then it's reassuring and predictable, and this gives us some degree of comfort in itself. You'll often see children playing with their hair or sucking their thumb at times of stress – it's similar to this.

The second is that when smokers are stressed and they light up a cigarette, they engage in other behaviours that really do reduce their stress and help them cope. For example, they get up, stop what they're doing, focus on something else, sit somewhere comfortable or stand outside. They take a break from whatever it is that's causing them stress or difficulty. Of course, the fact that they're smoking is incidental; these are exactly the same things that non-smokers do too – they're normal coping mechanisms, and you certainly don't need to smoke to do them.

It's inevitable that at some point when someone has stopped smoking they will experience some stressful circumstance and need to cope with this. As you know, non-smokers cope with life perfectly well, so clearly there are other coping mechanisms that don't rely on cigarettes. So, the next exercise is designed to get you to start thinking about alternative coping strategies.

EXERCISE 12: NEW WAYS OF COPING

Look back at the diary you made in Exercise 4 (page 60) and look at the cigarettes you smoked. Identify those that you smoked because you felt you needed them to cope. Write a list of the events that were happening at the time – the stressful, upsetting, anxious or difficult events that occurred. Maybe you were on the phone to the bank, or had just had a row with someone. It might be something quite small, like having to think how to word a tricky email to someone or the prospect of going somewhere or doing something new.

Now consider how else you might have coped with the stress. Write down a list of these alternative strategies. They might include taking a deep breath, relaxing or daydreaming, reading an article in a magazine, getting up from your desk for a few minutes and making some tea, going to the shop, phoning a friend, watching a stupid video of a cat getting chased by a rabbit on YouTube. It doesn't really matter; they will all inevitably be forms of removing yourself temporarily from the situation, giving yourself a bit of a break, allowing you to think through the problem and return to whatever it was afresh. This is precisely what all non-smokers do and it works perfectly well for them.

If you feel a bit stuck on this exercise, then I want you to show the list to a friend who doesn't smoke. Ask them what they would have done in that situation to cope. I can guarantee that the answer won't be that they'd start up smoking!

24
Cues

Smoking is a behaviour that, because of the frequency with which people do it, easily becomes engrained into their day-to-day lives. We learn to associate certain situations with a certain behaviour – in this case, smoking. This is called 'conditioning'. Part of becoming free from cigarettes is identifying and challenging this engrained behaviour, and the triggers and associations that our minds have made with it. To do this, you will need to carefully think about how, why and when you are prompted to smoke.

You may feel like you just smoke when you fancy it – but that's not the case. You might have a bag of crisps when you fancy it, but you don't do that 20 times a day, and you don't panic if you realise that you've run out of crisps. Smoking is easily associated with places, times, feelings and people. When exposed to these cues, smokers are conditioned to reach for their cigarettes and light up.

Below is an exercise to explore this in detail and help you understand the cues that have been set up in your mind in relation to smoking. It's similar to Exercise 4, your one-day smoking diary, but goes into a little more detail. This time though, it's the detail that's more important than simply the time.

EXERCISE 13: THINKING ABOUT YOUR SMOKING DIARY

This exercise looks at one day's worth of smoking. Preferably it should be a day that represents a standard day in your life, such as a usual workday (so not a day when you're going to a wedding or having an operation, for example, or if some other unusual event is happening). Draw a table with six columns and fill it out for each cigarette you have during this day. The table should have the following headings at the top:

Time	Location	People	Thoughts	Feelings	Other

Each time you smoke a cigarette, fill out a row in the table. So, for example, your first cigarette of the day might look something like this:

Time	Location	People	Thoughts	Feelings	Other
7:30am	Kitchen table	Alone	Stressed about work meeting	Nervous	Had with cup of coffee

Do the same for each cigarette so that, by the end of the day, you have a list of times, and, for each time, you have a list of locations, people, thoughts and feelings. Under the 'other' category, put in anything else that's relevant to the cigarette – any triggers or associations you had.

Once you have done this, sit down the following day and look carefully at the list. Firstly look at the locations that the smoking occurred in. There will inevitably be places where you smoke more than others. Look at the thoughts and feelings that accompany each cigarette. In Chapter 37 we will look at the importance of avoiding all these triggers and what you can do to change your routine to ensure that these triggers, associations and cues are minimised. But for now, just examine the list to try to understand the cues and triggers that are important for your smoking.

25
Timeline

I have heard many people say to me that they wished they'd stopped smoking when they were younger, but now that they've been smoking too long they don't see the point in stopping. The damage has already been done. You might feel the same way, and, if so, I'm sure this makes you feel, deep down, despondent and depressed. Don't worry. It's common for smokers to feel like this, but this thinking is flawed for two reasons.

The first reason is that underlying it remains the belief that smoking actually does something for you, when it does not. It gives you absolutely nothing and therefore it doesn't matter how old you are, so why not free yourself from this illusion? Who wants to end their lives having been duped by a heartless, manipulative and cynical industry that is happy to take thousands of pounds of your money and doesn't give a hoot that its products are killing you. What slave would say, even on their deathbed, 'Oh, don't worry about freeing me. I've been a slave so long, I might as well die one.' No, it doesn't matter if you're 20 or 120, it's never too late to free yourself. The feeling of changing your understanding about your relationship with cigarettes and realising that you no longer need them is one of the greatest feelings possible. It is truly exhilarating when a smoker realises that this thing that they thought they had to do, day in and day out, has finally gone and they have done it all by themselves. Realising the power of your mind to change your understanding of something is thrilling beyond words. I want everyone to experience that feeling.

The second reason is that, almost as soon as you stop smoking, you start to get benefits, so it's never too late to stop. This is illustrated in the below timeline, which shows the health benefits after you stop smoking.

After you've stopped for:

- **20 minutes:** Your blood pressure and heart rate will start to drop back towards normal levels.
- **2 hours:** Your heart rate and blood pressure have now decreased to normal levels. The peripheral circulation – that's the small blood vessels that feed your skin, arms and legs – starts to improve. More oxygen starts to get to your fingers and toes. It might surprise you to know that this is also the peak time for nicotine cravings. How many times have you gone for two hours without a cigarette? This is as bad as it gets.
- **8 hours:** The nicotine levels in your body have reduced by 90 per cent.
- **12 hours:** Your blood is starting to get rid of the highly toxic chemical carbon monoxide that is in cigarette smoke. (This nasty chemical reduces the amount of oxygen in your red blood cells and makes you feel lethargic – for more

on this, see Chapter 27). After only 12 hours, the carbon monoxide levels in your body are already dropping and your levels of oxygen are increasing.

- **24 hours:** It's only been a day and already your risk of having a heart attack is dropping. Smokers are 70 per cent more likely to have a heart attack than non-smokers but your risk is now starting to decrease.

- **48 hours:** As we discussed earlier, smoking kills the cells involved in smell and taste, but, after just two days, these cells start to regrow, meaning that you'll start to appreciate your food more. It's like going from tasting and smelling in black and white to glorious Technicolor.

- **72 hours:** By now, the nicotine has completely left the body. As a result of this, people start to experience more frequent withdrawals, but remember two things. Firstly, each withdrawal is mild – the actual pang for a cigarette quickly passes and isn't any more intense than the feeling you had after two hours without a cigarette. Because they happen more frequently at this point though, people start to panic and wonder if they'll ever be free of them. This is why lots of people relapse at this point. But the second thing to remember is that from this day onwards, it gets easier. It will never be as bad as this day, because every day from now onwards, your nicotine receptors are being 'down-regulated' – that is, they are being slowly destroyed because you're no longer using them (see page 52 to refresh your memory on this). Over the coming weeks, the body will destroy all the excess nicotine receptors that you've made while smoking and you'll return to normal levels, as if you never smoked. Remember the analogy of the little squawking baby birds sitting in a nest, crying out to be fed (page 51)? Today they are crying out more frequently, but, because there's no food for them, they will start to die off from now onwards. The lungs are also starting to relax so that breathing becomes easier.

- **4 days:** Around this time, people sometimes start to experience a cough. This seems strange that shortly after you stop smoking you start coughing. Surely that's not right? Well, the reason is both wonderful and awful in equal measure. It's awful because it's another example of what cigarette smoke does to the body, but wonderful because it also shows how incredible the body is at repairing itself.

  The cough is down to the fact that there are millions of tiny hairs, called cilia, that line the tubes to the lungs. These hairs have an incredibly important function for the lungs: they ensure the lungs remain clean and clear. They do this by constantly moving in a carefully coordinated motion – a bit like a Mexican wave at a football match – and this wafts any tiny particles of dust that might have been inhaled upwards and out of the lung. Smoking, however, kills these tiny cilia. I remember at medical school looking at the airways of smokers and non-smokers under the microscope. In the non-smoker, you could see the millions and millions of tiny little hairs lining the tube. In the smoker, it was completely smooth. After a few days without smoking though, your cilia start to grow back, and, boy, do they have some work to catch up on. Not only has all the dust and rubbish from the air collected in the lungs, but all the muck from the cigarettes that has been inhaled needs to be shifted out of the lungs too. As your lungs start to clear themselves, this can sometimes cause a cough, as your body desperately tries to bring up all the debris. It's irritating but usually will only last a week or two – and just think of what it's actually doing. Your body is finally able to spring-clean your lungs, getting rid of all the muck that has been stuck down there for years.

As an aside, this is different to the cough that smokers have – the 'smoker's cough' – which is caused by the muck in your lungs irritating and inflaming the delicate lung tissues. With a smoker's cough, the only way to get this muck, and the mucus that the lung produces in response to it, out of the lung, is to cough it up – because the cilia have been killed off and the lung has no other means of removing it.

- **5–8 days:** During this period, your body continues to repair itself and the nicotine receptors in your brain continue being destroyed. On average, people experience three pangs of withdrawal a day. The maximum amount of time they last is three minutes, but remember: they are mild and a sign that the body is ridding itself of the excess nicotine receptors and returning to normal.

- **10 days:** By this stage, the average person reports only two withdrawal pangs a day, usually lasting less than a minute. Your blood circulation to your teeth and gums has now returned to normal. Smile!

- **2 weeks:** Your exercise tolerance and general fitness is now significantly improved and your lungs have usually cleared themselves of most of the debris that has been stuck down there. The result is that people notice their breathing starts to improve. Also, people's skin starts to improve around this time. Withdrawal symptoms have usually dissipated by this point too.

- **4 weeks:** As the cilia in your lungs continue to regrow, so your risk of chest infections decreases.
- **3 months:** The average life span of a red blood cell is 3 months, so now all of your red blood cells that were damaged by the carbon monoxide in cigarette smoke have been replaced with healthy new red blood cells. Your lung capacity increases by up to 30 per cent. By now, the amount of nicotine receptors in the brain are at normal levels.
- **9 months:** By this time, your lungs have begun to repair themselves. Your cilia are now fully functioning, and all the muck in your lungs has been cleared.
- **1 year:** Your risk of heart disease has now decreased by 50 per cent compared to a smoker.
- **5 years:** Your risk of having a stroke is now back to the level of someone who has never smoked. Your risk of dying of lung, oesophageal, throat and mouth cancer is now half that of a smoker. Your risk of developing diabetes is now the same as a non-smoker.
- **10 years:** Your risk of dying of lung cancer is now reduced to that of someone who has never smoked.
- **13 years:** The average smoker who lives to 75 years old has six fewer teeth than a non-smoker. But, by 13 years after stopping, your risk of losing teeth is the same as someone who has never smoked.

- **15 years:** Your risk of heart disease is back to the level of someone who has never smoked. This means that you'll no longer be at an increased risk of conditions like a heart attack, coronary heart disease or angina. Your risk of pancreatic cancer has also dropped to that of someone who has never smoked.

So, from just a few minutes after you stop smoking, the body is already starting to repair itself and undo the damage that tobacco has done. I find it incredible that the body is able to do this – and that all we have to do is allow it to get on with it.

26
Weight worries

Weight gain after stopping smoking is a real concern that I've heard from lots of patients, and, although we've touched upon this in Chapter 15, it's worth discussing again in detail. It's strange that, given the amount of worry this generates, it isn't discussed in more depth by doctors and those involved in helping people quit smoking. The standard recommendation, if it's thought about at all, is to help smokers go on a diet when they quit smoking. This is, in my mind, totally wrong-headed and can be entirely counterproductive. What a diet does is merely emphasise that smoking had some positive benefit, placing further pressure and changes on the person who has quit. By going on a diet the former smoker is trying to change two different behaviours and this is a big undertaking. Research has shown that people who try to quit smoking and also diet at the same time are more likely to relapse.

The first thing to understand is the relationship between food, weight and cigarettes. There are a lot of myths surrounding this, some of which have been perpetuated by the tobacco industry. As early as the 1930s, cigarettes were promoted as a good tool for losing weight and keeping slim. It's important to understand the truth about how smoking does and doesn't affect body weight. Remember, body weight is determined by the number of calories consumed compared to the number of calories expended. Weight gain occurs when someone consumes more calories than they expend. The excess calories that aren't used are stored by the body as fat. Nicotine very briefly increases the smoker's metabolism, meaning that in theory they burn off calories slightly faster. In truth though, this effect is very minimal and so it can't be said to be a diet aid in any way. Studies have shown that the effect of smoking on metabolism is so small that it isn't able to explain the weight gain that some smokers report when they stop. Studies have also shown that nicotine also very slightly decreases the amount of food that smokers eat because it helps to prolong the feeling of fullness after a meal. It should be emphasised that this is only a small effect and doesn't last long, so in reality it has a negligible effect on keeping smokers slimmer compared to non-smokers. As with lots of aspects of smoking, these effects have been blown up out of all proportion and often act as a barrier for the smoker who is thinking of quitting.

Having said this, it is true that some smokers do put on weight when they stop. There are several reasons for this, although it is not that the cigarettes were acting as some sort of dieting aid. When people stop smoking they often, unless they have addressed this beforehand, feel that they have deprived themselves of something. In order to counteract this, they often indulge in other things instead, to offset the feelings of deprivation by no longer smoking. This means they snack more and treat themselves to things that they previously would not have eaten. They might also drink more alcohol to replace the cigarettes they would have smoked, and alcohol has a lot of calories in it. Research has shown that the average person who stops smoking gains about 4 kilograms, mainly through snacking. So, for people who have recently quit without addressing the psychological aspect of their addiction, they are in a type of mourning for the cigarettes and compensate for this by eating more. And if you take in more calories than you expend then you'll put on weight.

Part of this can be offset by increased physical activity. Because of the physical impact of smoking on people's exercise tolerance, most smokers are quite sedentary and tend not to exercise very much, or at least not compared to those who do not smoke. Many people find that when they quit smoking, their health begins to quite rapidly improve and they can then take up more exercise. It's important to consider this as it will not only provide a good distraction and new focus when you quit smoking, but also it will increase your metabolism and make you burn off extra calories. When I stopped smoking I was very mindful of this and so had booked in with a personal trainer for immediately after I stopped. I went to the gym three times a week with the trainer for a few months to ensure that I was exercising regularly and pushing myself as much as possible. The result of this was I actually lost a bit of weight after stopping smoking. Doing exercise also shows you how quickly your body is recovering from the effects of smoking, and this can act as a great motivator. You don't have to go to the gym if you don't fancy it – go for a 15-minute run when you get back from work, or walk or cycle to and from work or similar.

Weight gain is a small price to pay for the enormous health benefits of stopping smoking. Even though being overweight is associated with health problems, these pale into insignificance compared to the risks associated with smoking. But both you and I know that, really, people aren't thinking about the health aspect of weight gain when they worry about this in relation to stopping smoking. It's the physical aspect of it – people don't want to put on weight for aesthetic reasons. The counterpoint to this is that stopping smoking will improve your physical appearance beyond belief. You'll have better skin, hair and teeth, and you won't smell (for more on this, see the next chapter).

Even if you do put on weight, you'll still be much more attractive. But you don't actually have to put on weight when you stop smoking.

Weight gain in people who have quit smoking is a sign that cigarettes still have a hold of them. They are replacing them with something because, somewhere deep within, they still feel that they are missing out on something. That's why it's important that this psychological aspect of addiction is addressed. Remember that you do not need to replace your cigarettes with anything because smoking gave you nothing in the first place. Go back to your notes on Exercise 9 (page 91) to remind yourself of the illogical thinking patterns that were underpinning your understanding of smoking.

In much the same way as we have done with cigarettes, let's now look at some of the myths and misunderstandings you might have about smoking and weight, and let's consider alternative ways of understanding these thoughts:

Unhelpful thoughts:	Alternative, helpful thoughts:
Smoking helps me eat less during a meal.	Cigarettes are not a real appetite suppressant and I do not need to eat more to compensate for not smoking.
Smoking helps to stop me snacking.	Smoking does not provide me with anything and doesn't affect my need for food in any way. I do not need to start eating lots because I'm not replacing anything. If I feel peckish, I can snack in the same way as I did before stopping smoking.
In the past I've quit and gained weight and then started smoking again. I can't afford to put on any more weight.	In the past I hadn't addressed the psychological aspect of my addiction. I am now doing this and realise that I do not have to substitute cigarettes with food because cigarettes gave me nothing.
I can have a cigarette instead of dessert.	Although in the past I might have smoked instead of having a dessert, I can do other things at the end of the meal, such as have coffee or tea, chew gum, drink mineral water or eat some fruit. In fact, I'm used to not having a dessert so why would I start now?
I must restrict my diet when I stop smoking to avoid putting on weight.	In order to maintain my current weight, I simply need to eat exactly the same as I did when I was smoking. Just because I've stopped smoking doesn't mean I have to eat more. But it also doesn't mean I have to eat any less.

I need to treat myself in order to feel happy now that I've stopped smoking.	Smoking was not a treat for me. It was killing me and causing countless physical problems. I had fallen into a trap with smoking and I've now climbed out of that trap. I am free from smoking and feel happier and healthier because of it. I do not need to substitute food for cigarettes.
Smoking helps keep me thin and I feel attractive when I'm thin.	Smoking in itself did not keep me thin. I'm lots more attractive now that I don't smoke.

Some smokers are overweight to start with and, now that they have begun to address their smoking, they also want to address their weight. If this is you, that is great, but you should take things slowly, one step at a time. Don't rush things. Stopping smoking requires a lot of mental energy to change your relationship with cigarettes and the grip you feel they have on you. It is best to wait about six months after quitting smoking before considering addressing any weight concerns. Smoking has the most serious health implications so this should be addressed first.

27
Physical benefits of not smoking

I started off this book by saying that I wasn't going to dwell on the physical health problems associated with smoking, because we all know them. This is true, and certainly, as a way of stopping smoking on its own, banging on about the impact on our health doesn't do much good. But, having said that, before we move on to the next part of the book and prepare for quitting, it's useful to remind ourselves of some of the effects that smoking does have on our physical health. This is because smokers try to minimise these effects, when, in fact, it's a large part of why so many smokers deep down want to stop. So please do read through this section carefully and don't skim it. It's not a lecture and you might be pleasantly surprised by the fact that, no matter how long you've been smoking, it's not too late to stop some of the damage that cigarettes can do.

We all know that smoking causes cancer. It's not just lung cancer. It also causes bowel cancer, stomach cancer, bladder cancer and mouth cancer. It also causes heart disease. This can lead to strokes and bad circulation that can result in leg amputations, blindness and so on. The list of problems goes on. All of this seems so far into the distance that it's all too easy for the smoker to put off thinking about them. It also all seems a bit catastrophic and terminal, and most people are in a perpetual state of denial about the fact that they're mortal and going to die at some point, so may easily ignore these warnings.

But there are some things that tend to resonate more with people than simply saying, 'You'll get cancer/have a stroke/heart attack.'

The first is for you men out there. Smoking makes you impotent. It's normal for the strength of erection to decrease as we age. But smoking accelerates this significantly. In fact, some studies have suggested that it has such a serious impact on erections that it's the number one cause of impotence in otherwise healthy men. Now I don't know about you, but I find the thought of doing something that gets rid of this ability horrifying. The good news is that once you stop smoking your erections will get stronger again. Even better: the sexual sensation improves and your orgasms will increase in intensity. This is because, in the smoker, the circulation to the penis and its nerves is impaired. When you stop smoking, the circulation improves and the nerves get more oxygen and nutrients and work better. Prepare to feel like an adolescent again (well, within reason).

For women, there is the fertility issue. Smoking is strongly linked to infertility and problems conceiving. If there were a substance that was put into tap water that made women have reduced fertility, there would be an outcry. If there were a food that was shown to make men impotent and women infertile, no one would touch it with a bargepole, and rightly so. You'd stand looking at it in the supermarket and think to yourself: what nutcase buys this? If you then, for some reason, tried it and realised that it smelled and tasted disgusting, you'd be disbelieving that anyone actually chose to eat it. And yet this is exactly the situation with cigarettes. But the brilliant news is that, from the moment you stop smoking, your fertility will start to improve. And, don't worry, it's not just men that have better sensitivity and orgasms when they stop smoking; the same thing happens in women, as the improved circulation means that they are more easily aroused and that their clitoris is more sensitive.

And for both men and women, smoking is ageing. You can tell a middle-aged smoker a mile off. They have sallow, grey, unhealthy-looking skin. They have more wrinkles than non-smokers. There isn't a face cream in the world that can improve wrinkles like stopping smoking. Smoking also dries the skin, and there's some evidence that it increases the chance of spots and acne. A recent study conducted in Italy suggested that smokers were four times more likely to have acne compared to non-smokers.

While we're on the topic of appearance, one thing many smokers fail to realise is the impact that smoking has on their teeth. I don't just mean that they look tobacco-stained, which of course they do. Because smoking affects the circulation – in particular, the small, fragile blood vessels – the gums don't get enough oxygen. This causes them to recede. In fact, smoking is one of the main reasons for gum recession. As the gum recedes, it exposes the sensitive part of the tooth that should normally be protected by the edge of the gum. The long-term effect is that there is less gum keeping the tooth in place, and the teeth can become loose and have to be removed. Once the gum has started to recede, the only thing that can stop it progressing is stopping smoking. Despite being a doctor, I didn't appreciate this aspect of smoking until my dentist pointed it out one day and showed me how much my gums had receded already. I innocently asked what the long-term solution was. 'Dentures,' she replied as I stared at her in absolute horror. I'm sure it's no coincidence that shortly after this I stopped smoking. Don't worry though – as soon as you stop smoking, your gum health starts to improve. Since stopping smoking, my gum recession has also stopped – the same will happen for you.

The other thing that people often gloss over when thinking about the health benefits of not smoking is energy. I've never been a morning person and, in fact, hated the mornings. I felt sluggish and tired and groggy each morning regardless of what time I got up. I'd chosen jobs simply on the basis of what time I'd have to wake up in order to get there, I hated mornings that much. But then when I stopped smoking something truly unbelievable happened. After about two weeks I noticed that something had changed. Suddenly mornings weren't as bad as they always seemed to have been. In fact, mornings weren't that bad at all. I actually felt awake when I woke up, as opposed to feeling in a state of muddle-headedness and grogginess for the first hour. My thoughts were clearer and I felt brighter. It was such a dramatic change that other people even remarked on how alert I looked in the mornings.

The reason that smoking decreases your energy is that cigarette smoke contains in it, as well as nicotine, thousands of other chemicals that affect the body, one of which is carbon monoxide, which I mentioned briefly in Chapter 25. This nasty chemical binds to the red blood cells that carry oxygen to our cells. When combined with the decreased lung function also caused by smoking, this reduces the oxygen levels in the blood. Now, just as people who are being poisoned slowly by a dodgy boiler that is spewing out carbon monoxide into their flat complain of feeling tired and lethargic, so I had been deliberately poisoning myself with the same chemical (admittedly in smaller doses). It was like taking an anaesthetic each day. And the sad thing was I had been smoking for so long that I just assumed this is what mornings were like for everyone – I thought that feeling groggy and half asleep when you wake up was normal. Stopping smoking stops this gradual, insidious poisoning and means that, within just a few weeks, you start experiencing a new energy that you'd forgotten you ever had and that non-smokers take for granted. It's like being given an aspect of your life back you hadn't even realised had been taken from you.

PART FOUR

ACTION

In this section we're going to look at how to prepare for and to actually stop smoking. We will cover some of the practical things you can do to ready yourself for quitting and to make sure that you make it as easy as possible for yourself. This is important because, while the thoughts that underpin smoking need to be understood and tackled, it's also important to understand and prepare for triggers that might catch you off guard. There are also some exercises to help you keep focused and motivated as you move towards being smoke-free.

28
Preparing for action

We've seen how the mind plays tricks on smokers to justify behaviour that we know, deep within, is bad for us and wish we didn't do. We've also seen how, although it feels like smoking is important, it actually gives smokers nothing – and the only reason we smoke is because of the illusions and distortions that form the smoking trap we have fallen into. But how do you actually turn this knowledge into action? There is always a risk that smokers will fall back on the 'one day' argument (see Chapter 22) as an attempt to put off actually stopping. To move from being a smoker to a non-smoker, you need, not just an understanding of the thought patterns that maintain your smoking behaviour, but also some practical planning. The rest of this book will look at this aspect of stopping smoking.

To mentally prepare yourself for actually moving into the action phase of behaviour change, I want you to do the following brief exercise:

EXERCISE 14: RECAP

Look back over all of the previous exercises and remind yourself what you have learned from them. Remember the tricks that your mind has been playing on you in order to keep you smoking and help you to justify this to yourself. Go right back to the beginning when you listed all the things you thought you loved about smoking, through to the story you wrote about how you came to start smoking and the associations you had with it, and then to the list of reasons to continue smoking, through to the reasons to quit and your expanded smoking diary. If you skipped any of these exercises, then now is the time to do them.

29
Set a date

I said in Chapter 19 that the smoker will always find something in their life to put off stopping, and this is true. Life is full of stresses and, if you wait until you have absolutely no stress or difficulties, you are likely to be dead before this happens. Having said that, there are clearly better times to stop smoking than others, and a little preparation in this regard can help ensure you succeed. I'm not going to be too prescriptive with the exact date you choose, but it should be *within* two weeks of finishing this book and the exercises inside it. If you leave it any longer than that, you'll start to forget all the work you've done and everything you've learned about your relationship with cigarettes, and it will be harder for you.

So, get your diary or calendar, look at the next fortnight and pick a day. Remember that all the nicotine will have left your system by day three, so this is often the hardest day. Don't panic though; a bit of forward planning can make sure this day passes without you even really noticing it. Much of smoking is about cues, triggers and routine, so it's important that this is pre-empted and prepared for. We're going to make sure that as much of your usual routine – the routine that included cigarettes – is different to minimise the triggers.

Personally, I found stopping just before going on a holiday was very helpful. I spent the evening packing and getting ready, all along mentally preparing myself for the following day when I would become a non-smoker. It was quite exciting, although a little nerve-wracking too. I couldn't believe I was actually going to do it. I went outside just before midnight for my last cigarette and then went to bed. I got up the next day early in the morning and got a taxi to the airport and, before I realised it, it was the afternoon, I hadn't had a cigarette and I was sitting on a sun lounger by a rooftop pool in a hotel overlooking Barcelona. It was so peaceful and lovely and different to my usual day, it barely even registered that I wasn't smoking. Whenever the thoughts of cigarettes entered my head, I thought to myself: 'That was something I used to do. I don't do that now,' and a little buzz of excitement went through me.

That's not to say that there weren't times when I wasn't tempted to smoke. This was a behaviour I had done for the majority of my life; it was never going to be a complete walk in the park. In fact, I'd only been sitting on the sun lounger for a few hours when my decision to stop smoking was tested. The man lying next to me turned and asked me for a light. I instinctively went to put my hand in my pocket, before remembering that I no longer smoked. I turned to the man to say that I was a non-smoker and realised it was George Michael. Of all the bloody days to become a non-smoker, I thought to myself. Any hope of sitting there sharing a cigarette with him while he sang 'Careless Whisper' was scuppered. But I then reminded myself that he had only recently been in a hospital and nearly died. As I lay back down on the lounger, it occurred to me that he may be infinitely cool and a very talented singer but, despite nearly dying, he was still stuck in the trap that I had managed to climb out of. I actually ended up feeling quite sorry for him (and a little bit gutted that he hadn't become my new best friend).

So, you might want to consider going away somewhere if you can arrange it (with cameos from A-list celebrities optional), just to break the usual routine to get you over the initial strangeness of not smoking. Remember, though, that this only postpones, rather than fully avoids, the triggers that are there in your day-to-day life. Certainly they will be easier to deal with when you've had a few days, or even longer, of being smoke-free, but you must still prepare for being confronted with situations when you would have previously smoked on your return home. Chapter 37 will help you prepare for facing these kind of triggers.

If you can't take a holiday then don't worry. You will need to choose a day that allows for you to change your routine to some degree though. On the day you stop smoking, don't worry if you still have cigarettes in the packet, just throw them away. This isn't a waste – they are hateful, disgusting, misery-making objects that are ruining your life and trapping you in a behaviour you want to stop. Chuck them out with glee. Don't use the few sitting in the packet as an excuse to keep smoking.

To prepare yourself for what your first few days are going to be like, I want you to do the following exercise:

EXERCISE 15: VISUALISE YOUR FIRST DAYS AS A NON-SMOKER

Go back to Exercise 7 (page 71), when you looked at your diary or calendar and imagined a day in the future and what it would be like if you were a non-smoker. Now, I want you to do the same thing but for the days immediately after your quit day. Think about where you'll be and what you'll be doing, the people you will meet and the challenges you'll face on those days. I want you to go through them in as much detail as you can, imagining yourself as a non-smoker. Think about alternative strategies to smoking for dealing with the problems or situations you might face on those days. If you get stuck, go back to some of the answers you came up with in Exercise 12 (page 116).

It should be noted that there is some evidence that for some women their menstrual cycle is relevant for when they choose to quit. It is thought that women who stop smoking during the first half of their menstrual cycle (days 1–14, the 'follicular phase') find it slightly easier compared to women who quit during the second half of their cycle (days 15–28, the 'luteal phase'). The evidence isn't completely conclusive, and no one is really quite sure why it might play a part, but it's thought that it's possibly because women who quit during the second phase also have to contend with premenstrual symptoms, which can mimic nicotine withdrawal symptoms, making the quitters believe the experience is worse. The general guide is that if you experience particularly bad premenstrual symptoms, then it's best to choose a quit day at the beginning of your cycle.

30
Detoxify your house

From now on until your quit day, I want you to stop smoking in the house. It's fine – you can still smoke as much as you want, just not in your house. There are three reasons for this. Firstly, it makes things a little more inconvenient. You have to make an active decision to smoke, rather than just mindlessly lighting up. You can take this book with you outside if you want, so you can still smoke and read. Secondly, doing this clears your house of the smell, which might act as a trigger. Finally, it shows that you are in control of when you smoke. This also goes for the car if you smoke in there too. From now on, I only want you to smoke outdoors. I don't care if it's raining – use an umbrella if you have to.

31
Getting rid of smoking paraphernalia

Next, I want you to throw away all your lighters and ashtrays. Remember that box of matches I wanted you to get when you first started reading this book? Well, now you know what they were for. From now on, use only the matches to light your cigarettes. They're easier to throw away and are less associated with cigarettes than lighters. Ashtrays and lighters are visual prompts that, if you have them lying around your house, will prompt you to want a cigarette. They are also the paraphernalia of committed smokers, and therefore must go. I also want you to go through all your bags, coat pockets, drawers and down the back of the sofa to make sure you don't have any extra cigarettes hanging around or lighters that you might come across after your quit date.

The one issue with this piece of advice is that you might have a nice lighter. I had a very expensive lighter that was given to me by a friend. It was worth several hundred pounds, and it felt a shame to simply throw this away. Likewise, it didn't feel right to sell it, as then I was just giving the problem of what to do with a valuable lighter when you no longer wanted to smoke to someone else. In the end I gave it to a non-smoker friend to look after while I stopped smoking and a few months later got it back; now I just use it to light candles. Everything else, though, I threw away, and you should too.

32
Reducing before stopping

Some people like the idea of reducing the number of cigarettes they smoke before actually stopping them. I've deliberately not advocated this technique in this book because the whole point of a CBT approach to smoking is to challenge the way we think about smoking and to bring about a change in the relationships with cigarettes that way. Most people who undergo this sort of approach find that, as they progress through it, the desire to smoke lessens anyway. If this happens and you find yourself naturally smoking less, then that is fine and, for goodness' sake, don't force yourself to smoke.

What tends to happen though to people who simply reduce the amount they smoke without undergoing any psychological work is that they manage to cut down for a time, while their motivation to do so is high, but they still feel like they are denying themselves something. Soon something happens that is stressful or difficult and, because they hadn't fully explored the psychological dimension of their addiction, they resort to the only coping strategy they know – smoking. And so they increase back up to the same number they were on previously.

All that's happened is that they've had a few weeks of feeling virtuous, tinged with the feeling that ultimately they were sacrificing something, and then they've had the crushing blow of relapsing back to the same number. Even if you do a carefully planned reduction and stick to it, my personal feeling is that you are unnecessarily drawing out the process. You want the nicotine out of your system as soon as possible so that the receptors in your brain can start to die back.

33
Tell a friend

Telling people you are planning on stopping smoking is a mixed bag. On one hand, it's good to get encouragement and support from people. On the other hand, it can backfire because, depending on who you tell, it can put excessive pressure on you, which is rather counterproductive. The last thing you want is to feel that your entire family, for example, are breathing down your neck and checking you've not relapsed.

Alternatively, if you tell some people – and by some people, I mean some smokers – they will probably feel overwhelmed by guilt that *they* are not stopping and jealousy that you are. You must be aware of this happening and prepare for it. When I first stopped smoking I was really astonished by how many people I considered good friends tried to get me to start up smoking again. They were being entirely selfish because they hated that yet another one of their number was abandoning them and joining the smoke-free brigade. Smokers are increasingly isolated and alone, so when one of their own leaves, they don't like it. They get scared because they worry that they will have to stop smoking too and they are not prepared for this. It exacerbates the fear that all smokers feel about quitting, and this often causes them to react in a surprisingly selfish and callous way.

That's not to say all smokers are the same as this – some of my friends who continued smoking were incredibly supportive and kept on telling me how proud they were of what I had done. About a week after stopping smoking I was drunk in a bar and found a rather crushed cigarette in the top pocket of the jacket I was wearing. I looked at it momentarily, rather tempted. Before I could do anything about it, a friend who at the time was a committed smoker (and has since quit), saw me with it in my hand from across the room, dashed over and jumped on my back to snatch it off me before snapping it in half. Even though she smoked, she was desperate for me to succeed in quitting. That's a proper friend.

So, think carefully about who you tell that you are planning on quitting, but be in no doubt that telling at least someone can be a great support. Former smokers – providing they haven't turned into those ex-smokers we talked about in Chapter 4, who are just going to nag you to stop smoking – are often the best because they understand the pitfalls, and what will help, better than someone who has never smoked.

34
Write a contract

When you've found at least one person who you think will support you in your quest to stop smoking, write up a contract to yourself and ask them to witness it. This might sound a bit daft, but writing a contract puts down in black and white your commitment to stop smoking and helps you identify the key reasons why you are going to stop.

To write your contract, go back to Exercise 11 (page 112) and use your golden three reasons to quit to fill out the quitting contract in the exercise below. You can add in some more supplementary reasons for deciding to stop smoking by looking back at your quit list from Exercise 6 (page 68) if you want to. Carry your contract with you in your wallet or purse as a reminder to you as to why you wanted to stop smoking when you have the urge to relapse. Of course, no one is going to get sued if you break this contract but seeing your commitment written down is a powerful way of cementing your determination to stop. I've written a template contract below, but feel free to tweak the wording as you see fit:

EXERCISE 16: YOUR QUITTING CONTRACT

Stopping smoking is going to make me happier, richer and healthier. I have decided that I am going to free myself from the trap I have fallen into, and I now realise that smoking gives me nothing. Everything that I thought it gave me was a trick of the mind.

Therefore, I (insert name) am going to stop smoking on (insert date).

My main reasons for deciding to stop smoking are:
1.   2.   3.

It is going to change my life because:
1.   2.   3.

The worst things about smoking that I will be happy to rid myself of include:
1.   2.   3.

If I need support, I can contact the following person: (insert name)

Signature: Date:

Witness: Date:

35
Money talks

We haven't discussed the amount of money the smoker quite literally sends up in smoke every day. Over the past few years the cost of cigarettes has rocketed and is inevitably going to continue to increase. I remember vaguely thinking about this but never really allowing myself to dwell on the vast amount of money I was wasting – after all, I thought I loved smoking and therefore this was a small price to pay for something I loved. But I do remember vaguely thinking that when I couldn't get any change from a £5 note for a packet of cigarettes, I'd stop. Huh! Yet again, this was a delay tactic of my mind to prevent me from having to confront the need to stop smoking, just as I had done by saying to myself that I'd stop when I was 30. Of course, before I knew it I was spending £6, then £7, on a packet.

I remember when I first started smoking and a packet of cigarettes cost under £2.50. At the time of writing, I just popped out to the shops to check and they are now at nearly £9. I can guarantee that, before too long, they will be over £10. That's an increase of 400 per cent. At what point will it become too expensive for you? At what point will you realise that you are wasting a fortune on something that gives you absolutely nothing except the possibility of horrible, crippling disease?

There's some good evidence to show that when people are confronted with the amount of money they spend each year on cigarettes, this can be a good motivator to stop. So, the next exercise is simple:

EXERCISE 17: AN EXPENSIVE ADDICTION

Work out the amount of money you spend each year on cigarettes. Take the amount of money you spend a day and multiply this by 365. So, for the average pack-a-day smoker, this would be:

- £9 x 7 = £63 a week
- That's £273 a month
- That's £3,276 a year

Now that's a lot of money. Over the course of 10 years, that would be over £30,000 – and that's not even allowing for any further increase in price.

I'm aware that this is a bit abstract. People will often say: imagine all the things you could spend that money on! But, in reality, this isn't how people manage their finances. It acts as a fairly good motivator, but as the weeks and months go by, you'll just be spending it on other things. I was determined this wasn't going to happen to me, because I wanted to be able to show myself a month, six months, a year down the line that the impact that this one decision – this decision to stop smoking – had had on my finances. So, I opened up another bank account and set up a weekly direct debit for the amount of money I would have spent on cigarettes that week. It went from my regular bank account into this new bank account, and I just left it. Doing it this way meant that I never noticed the money leaving my account, just as I never really noticed the money I spent on cigarettes. Over the weeks and months, the money kept on trickling in and, periodically, I'd take it out and spend it on something completely frivolous or fun. I went on a weekend away to Paris with it, I bought a ludicrously overpriced designer belt, I bought a cashmere blanket, I had afternoon tea at a swanky London hotel, I got my teeth whitened. I deliberately used it to buy or do things that I'd never normally be able to justify spending my money on because I wanted to show myself, firstly, how much money I'd been wasting all that time on smoking and, secondly, how much fun I could have precisely because I wasn't smoking. I still have that bank account now and it's a source of great excitement and fun, as every few months I allow myself to dip into it and spend the money on whatever I want. I'd definitely recommend this for when you stop smoking. Seen a pair of shoes for £500 that you can't even imagine ever buying? Well, they are only two months' worth of cigarettes. A top-of-the-range 50-inch plasma-screen TV? Don't smoke for four months and it's yours.

Set up a separate bank account and you won't notice the money leaving your account each week, but you will notice the financial benefits, and it will hammer home what a waste of cash smoking is. The only rule is you can spend the money on absolutely **whatever** you want – you can't waste it any more than you would have done by spending it on cigarettes.

36
Nicotine replacement therapies or medications

Nicotine replacement therapy (often shortened to NRT) is a group of products that contain nicotine, and is used by doctors and pharmacists to help people stop smoking. The products used are usually chewing gum, patches, lozenges or sprays. They work by providing the body with a specific dose of nicotine when taken. The idea is that the dose in the product is then gradually reduced over time so that the person is gently weaned off the nicotine.

Along with NRT, there are two medications that are sometimes prescribed to help people stop smoking: Zyban and Champix. They don't contain nicotine but work by decreasing the desire to smoke while the patient takes them.

Zyban is the brand name for the drug bupropion. This was initially marketed as an antidepressant but patients began reporting that, while taking it, they no longer wanted to smoke, so it was soon rebranded as a smoking-cessation medication.

It's not clear exactly how it works, but it is thought that it acts on chemicals in the brain (known as neurotransmitters). The usual regime is to take one tablet for six days, then increase this to one tablet twice a day, at least eight hours apart. The aim is to stop smoking on day eight of taking the medication. In total, people usually take the medication for a further seven weeks, meaning that in total the treatment lasts about two months. As with any medication, there can be side effects. These include difficulty sleeping, headaches, dry mouth, feeling sick, feeling shaky or agitated and constipation. It's also not suitable for everyone. It can interact with a long list of other medications and is often not prescribed to people who are breastfeeding, have problems with their liver or kidneys, a history of eating disorders or other mental-health problems, are diabetic, have seizures or high blood pressure or some skin problems. It's therefore important that, if you do decide to take this medication, you make sure the person prescribing it is aware of your medical history and what medications, if any, that you currently take. You should also make sure you take it exactly as instructed to by the doctor.

This is the same for the other medication that is sometimes prescribed, called Champix. This is the brand name for the drug varenicline. It works in an interesting way. Although it does not contain nicotine, it works on those nicotine receptors in the brain that we mentioned in Chapter 8. It binds to these receptors and therefore produces an effect that relieves withdrawals but also – and this is the clever bit – it stays on the receptor for a bit, meaning that it blocks any nicotine from smoke that's inhaled from getting to the receptor and producing an effect. This means that when the smoker smokes, they get no sense of reward from the cigarette. The dose is typically increased gradually in the first week of treatment and then taken twice a day for 12 weeks. The plan is for the smoker to stop smoking one week into the treatment course, when the concentration of the drug is at its optimum. If you remain smoke-free after the 12-week course, then sometimes the doctor may prescribe another course of treatment for up to a further 12 weeks in consultation with the patient and how they feel. Again, it can have side effects such as sleep problems, strange dreams, nausea and headaches. And, again, it's not suitable for everyone, with doctors only prescribing it with caution in people with kidney or heart problems, a history of mental illness or epilepsy.

Both of these medications can affect your ability to drive or use heavy machinery, and so people should refrain from doing so until they know how the medications affect them. The person prescribing the medication goes through all this in detail, though.

With both NRTs and medications, the decision whether or not to use them is entirely up to you. As I said at the beginning of this book, I tried every type of NRT on the market and none of them worked for me. They didn't address my feelings around cigarettes and so, as a result, it felt too much like I was denying myself something I loved. Despite my personal experiences, I have no objections to you trying NRTs or smoking-cessation medications. Some stop-smoking books prohibit you from these kind of products, but I think it's important that you should be able to use whatever helps you give up smoking. I don't care what you do or try, providing it works and you free yourself from smoking. But this comes with one important word of caution:

> You must realise that NRT and stop-smoking medications do not address the psychological aspect of smoking. As mentioned earlier, this is actually the really tricky aspect of smoking.

With NRTs, there is no doubt that they can help people quit smoking. However, the initial studies that showed dramatic benefit in helping smokers quit were mostly funded by the manufacturers of these products, and subsequent studies have suggested that they might not be as effective as first thought. I suspect that this is because, although NRT replaces the nicotine that the smoker would otherwise get from a cigarette, it fails to take into account the emotional relationship that smokers have with cigarettes. While you can replace the nicotine, if you don't address your relationship with cigarettes, then you will risk becoming one of those ex-smokers I mentioned in Chapter 4. You will still love cigarettes and miss them. You might not relapse back into smoking, but you might be miserable and depressed by the fact that you no longer smoke, and that would be such a shame.

If you're thinking of using NRT, then spend some time researching each of the different options. Remember, if you give them a try and they don't work for you, it's not the end of the world – there are plenty of different types out there. Your GP or pharmacist can also help.

With Zyban and Champix, while they both reduce the physical urge to smoke, they again do not significantly address the psychological effects. If the physical addiction were all there was to smoking, then the success rates for both of these medications would be 100 per cent, and they are not. Studies have shown that both have success rates of about 20 per cent, so for the other 80 per cent who relapse on these medications and start smoking again it clearly wasn't the whole answer.

So, by all means take Zyban or Champix if you want, and if the prescriber is happy to give one of them to you, but be aware that they can only ever be *part* of the answer to stopping smoking. You might find that, when you have addressed the psychological aspect of your addiction, the physical side is so insignificant and pathetic that you won't even need anything to help with this.

What I want to emphasise is that you can still use this book to address the psychological aspects of smoking whether or not you choose to use NRT, Zyban or Champix.

37

Avoiding triggers and breaking routines

Triggers for smoking take the form of places, situations, thoughts and objects. All of these are closely interrelated. So, sitting in the morning, drinking coffee and feeling stressed about going to work has all the components of this:

Time	Location	Thoughts	Other
7:30am	Kitchen table	Stressed about work	Had with cup of coffee

Make sure you are aware of the triggers that are present in your day – the times when you would normally smoke – and ensure that you do everything you can to avoid these. While you can't avoid all object triggers, like coffee, there are some such as lighters and ashtrays that you can avoid, which is why I emphasised in Chapter 31 the importance of getting rid of these before you stop. You could also try having your morning coffee, for example, in a coffee shop, where you can't smoke anyway.

We have seen how there are numerous triggers that cause smokers to light up and you've identified some of these yourself in Exercise 13 (page 119). When you decide to stop smoking, it's important to try to foresee these triggers and avoid them where possible. The best way to do this is to break your usual routine. This will help you avoid key places and situations you associate with smoking and get rid of the accidental temptations that would normally trigger you to light up.

This can actually be quite exciting as it's fun to change your daily routine every now and then anyway. I've mentioned going on holiday or having a break away from home and, while this can help the first few days, inevitably you'll have to return home and will find yourself surrounded by all the old triggers and associations again. So, even if you do stop smoking while on holiday, you'll still need to break routine when you get back.

The key to this strategy is changing the structure to your day. So perhaps try the following:

- Get up 10 minutes later than you would normally.
- Eat breakfast in a different place (either go out for breakfast or eat it in a different room) or change what you have for breakfast.
- Take a different route to work.
- Prepare for your breaks at work and make sure you have alternative plans to what you would normally do. Bring a book, magazine or download a game on to your mobile to play during breaks at work.

- Arrange to go out for lunch and, if possible, take your lunch break at a different time to usual.
- Plan your evenings carefully to ensure you're distracted and doing something different to what you would usually do.

You should aim to break your routine like this for at least two weeks.

38
When triggers remain

It is impossible to get rid of all the smoking triggers in your life. There will inevitably be times when you encounter a situation or thought or feeling that you associate with smoking. Similarly, there are bound to be situations or thoughts or feelings that in the past you would have dealt with by smoking. We've talked about coping and the need to find alternative strategies in Chapter 23, but I want you to think about this carefully now.

When you face a situation that needs a new strategy to replace smoking, the key considerations are:

- Remind yourself about why you have stopped smoking.
- Remind yourself that, although smoking feels like it helps you deal with difficulties, it does not.
- Remind yourself that the only reason it feels like smoking helps you cope is because it alleviates nicotine withdrawals – which smoking caused in the first place and perpetuates with every cigarette you smoke.

- Remind yourself that non-smokers cope with situations just as well as smokers, and there is no reason why you should have to use smoking as an artificial prop.
- Stay busy and plan your days carefully. Avoid boredom or not knowing what to do with yourself. Carry a book or some other activity with you.
- Practise relaxation techniques (we'll cover these in the next chapter).

39
Withdrawals

The thought of withdrawals is what keeps many smokers smoking. It is the fear of these that perpetuates the behaviour you are trying to stop. Stop being afraid.

Throughout this book I have emphasised that the withdrawals from nicotine are actually very mild, despite what you will have heard. It's actually the fear of not being able to smoke that makes withdrawals seem so much worse than they actually are. If you stop being afraid of no longer smoking, the withdrawals are a breeze. You will get them, but, remember, they are brief, mild and will pass. After day three of being smoke-free, the withdrawals will only get better and the whole thing usually only lasts two weeks. How you think about these episodes of craving will have a significant effect on how much they impact on you. Rather than seeing them as something scary or upsetting, view them as your body getting rid of the nicotine receptors that keep you addicted. After each craving, they will get less and less. So see each craving as a step towards being entirely free from cigarettes.

There are some practical things too that you can do to alleviate cravings when you have them. Firstly, I found that often I mistook being thirsty for a craving. Or, rather, when

I was thirsty, the sensation in the back of my throat was similar to the niggling craving for a cigarette, so it triggered an association with wanting a cigarette and brought on a craving. Drink plenty of water but also keep a bottle of iced water to hand. If you get a craving, take some sips of this iced water. Swallow the water hard so that it is squeezed against the back of your throat as you swallow. I found that the ice-cold sensation at the back of my throat as I did this was similar to the burn sensation of inhaling a cigarette, so I easily tricked my brain into forgetting that it thought it wanted a cigarette.

I also found that, when I had a sudden twinge of wanting to smoke, focusing very carefully on my breathing helped. I would then purse my lips very tight until just a tiny hole between my lips was left, and then draw the air in very quickly into my mouth, on to my tongue and down into my lungs. Sometimes I'd waggle the tip of my tongue inside my mouth in the stream of air I was creating as it went into my lungs. It looked completely weird, but the cold, thin stream of air hitting my tongue felt surprisingly invigorating and refreshing. It had a similar effect to the ice-cold water too on the back of the throat. It also reminded me how lovely cold, fresh air is compared to the hot, polluted fumes of a cigarette.

Most smokers who have quit report about three cravings a day for the first week, and then one or two for the next week or so. That's actually not very many at all. They can last around a minute, but most of them are actually very short – only a few seconds. The reason they can feel longer is because it causes the person to panic and become fearful about the sensation they are having so they start debating whether they should have a cigarette.

Relaxation techniques have been shown to be very useful in these circumstances, and below is an exercise to teach you how to do something called progressive muscle relaxation (PMR), which was developed in the 1920s by an American doctor. There are various videos to help with this on YouTube, but the basic principles are all the same and I've outlined it for you below. Practise this before your quit day so that it becomes second nature to you. It's intended to make you more aware of your body and what it feels like when it is tense. It also helps remind each muscle group how to relax and what this feels like. You can start off by doing this in bed before you go to sleep or lying in the bath while you get used to it.

EXERCISE 18: PROGRESSIVE MUSCLE RELAXATION

The goal of this exercise is to entirely relax your body, not to fall asleep.

Start by closing your eyes and taking slow, deep breaths in and out. Make sure you don't hold your breath through the exercise, but instead keep a steady, slow, deep pace in your breathing. In this exercise, you will sequentially relax and tense different muscles in your body. For each muscle, tense it for 10 seconds and then relax it for 10 seconds. While you are doing this, your attention should be entirely focused on the muscle group you are working on; all other muscles should remain entirely relaxed.

- **Scalp:** Tense your scalp and lift your eyebrows. Your forehead and scalp should be tense. Hold it for 10 seconds then entirely relax it for 10 seconds.
- **Face:** Screw up your eyes and nose as hard as you can. Hold it for 10 seconds then entirely relax it for 10 seconds.
- **Mouth:** Grimace your face so you show your teeth while clenching them hard. Hold it for 10 seconds then entirely relax it for 10 seconds.
- **Neck:** Push the bottom of your chin on to your chest until you can feel the pull. You should feel the tension in your neck and the back of your head. Hold it for 10 seconds then entirely relax it for 10 seconds.
- **Shoulders:** Scrunch your shoulders up to your ears. You should feel the tension in your shoulders. Hold it for 10 seconds then entirely relax it for 10 seconds.
- **Upper arms:** Push your upper arms against your rib cage as tightly as you can. Make sure you don't tense your lower arms as you do this. You should feel the tension in your upper arms, back and shoulders. Hold it for 10 seconds then entirely relax it for 10 seconds.

- **Lower arms:** Keeping your fingers relaxed, flex your wrist upwards so that they bend towards your forearms. You should feel the tension in your wrist and the backs of your forearms. Hold it for 10 seconds then entirely relax it for 10 seconds.
- **Hands:** Clench your fists while the rest of your arm remains entirely relaxed. Hold it for 10 seconds then entirely relax it for 10 seconds.
- **Shoulders:** Puff out your chest but, while you do this, arch your back and try to touch your shoulder blades together. Hold it for 10 seconds then entirely relax it for 10 seconds.
- **Abdomen:** Clench your abdominal muscles (you don't need a six-pack to do this – everyone has abdominal muscles), like when you are tensing when you're about to be sick or cough. Remember to keep breathing. Hold it for 10 seconds then entirely relax it for 10 seconds.
- **Thighs:** Squeeze your knees together and lift your legs up slightly, towards your chest. Keep your lower legs totally relaxed. Hold it for 10 seconds then entirely relax it for 10 seconds.
- **Lower legs:** Push your feet down as though you were on tiptoes. Feel the tension in the back of your lower leg. Hold it for 10 seconds then entirely relax it for 10 seconds. Then pull the feet up, towards the shin. Hold it for 10 seconds then entirely relax it for 10 seconds.

- **Feet:** Pull your feet inwards while splaying your toes upwards and outwards. Hold it for 10 seconds then entirely relax it for 10 seconds.

Remember that the cravings are brief and mild. When you have one, try saying a nursery rhyme to yourself (if you're at work, it's best to do this in your head rather than out loud, obviously). Say it slowly and clearly and visualise, if you can, what the nursery rhyme is about, as this will distract your mind. I did 'Mary had a little lamb' and whenever I got to the part 'its fleece was white as snow', I imagined white snow and fresh, bracing air and thought of my lungs clearing themselves of all that cancer-forming muck that I'd inhaled over the years. By the time you have finished the nursery rhyme, the cravings should have passed.

40
Dealing with relapse

This book should have shown you that the reasons you thought you had to continue smoking were not real. It should have helped you reprogramme your thinking about why you smoke and your relationship with cigarettes. That said, I'm a pragmatist and am aware that sometimes things don't go according to plan. People have moments of weakness when the rational part of their brain seems to lose control and they do things they regret. Despite all the hard work they have done, they find themselves having a cigarette. Rather than pretending this never happens, it's important to think about it.

Firstly, once you are a non-smoker, you must never try another cigarette. We have already seen in Chapter 8 that, because of an unfortunate quirk in your genes, your nicotine receptors are primed for you to become addicted to them. You will never be one of those people who can have the odd cigarette here and there. Often, after a few months into stopping smoking, people feel confident that they are now free from it. Their resolve slightly weakens because they have started to forget some of the things they learned about their thinking around smoking. They think, 'Well, one won't hurt.' There is also sometimes a perverse sense of wanting to prove to themselves that they are no longer addicted to nicotine and so, often when they are drunk or under pressure, they buckle under and try just one. This is fatal. You do not need to prove to yourself that you are not addicted to nicotine – the fact you no longer smoke is evidence enough. People who have never smoked are not addicted to nicotine but do not feel the need to prove this to themselves or other people by smoking one occasionally. Similarly, you never feel the need to prove to yourself that you are not addicted to heroin, for example, by trying it once. You know you're not addicted to it and you're jolly pleased you're not. Trying just one cigarette risks undoing all the psychological work that you have done.

However, if you do find that you have smoked, remember, it doesn't have to turn into a relapse. Time and time again, I have seen patients in my clinic who are addicted to heroin and relapsed. When I've asked them about it, they've explained that, for whatever reason, they found themselves trying it one more time, and then that opened the floodgates and, before they knew it, they were back to full-blown addiction. I'll say to you exactly what I say to them. Instead of viewing it as a relapse, view this as a slip-up. A mistake. Doing something once does not have to inevitably lead to you repeatedly doing it. This is highly important so I'm going to say it again. **Doing something once does not have to inevitably lead to you repeatedly doing it.**

Every time you light up a cigarette after that initial slip-up, you are guaranteeing that you will now revert to becoming a smoker. Don't start down this path. Learn from the mistake – identify what the trigger was that you hadn't prepared for, think about how you can avoid this in the future, wipe the slate clean and start afresh. One cigarette is not a reason to undo all your hard work. Go back over the book and look at the exercises again, particularly Exercises 6 and 9 (pages 68 and 91). You've slipped up, but you do not have to become a smoker again. You can choose to remain a non-smoker.

41
Q&As

Although this isn't strictly part of the CBT programme, there are two questions that I get asked a great deal, so I wanted to briefly answer them here, as you might be wondering about them too.

SHOULD YOU SWITCH TO ELECTRONIC CIGARETTES?

Over the past few years, the e-cigarette market has exploded. You can now buy them everywhere, from supermarkets to bars. They come in various shapes and sizes – with some looking like regular cigarettes (right down to having a brown speckled butt), while others look more like something out of *Star Trek* – but they all work on the same principle. They are a battery-powered device that, when sucked on, has a heating mechanism that is triggered to vaporise a liquid solution containing nicotine. This vapour – which looks like smoke but is odourless and quickly vanishes – is inhaled into the lungs and the nicotine is absorbed into the bloodstream. They often have a coloured light at the end that lights up when it is being sucked on, to mimic the glow of the tip of a cigarette when it is smoked.

They have actually been around for a long time – they were first patented in the 1960s, although were not widely used, and they vanished until the early 2000s, when a pharmacist in China honed the design, obtained a patent and began manufacturing them. By 2007 the first of these electronic, smokeless cigarettes was being exported. Since then, their popularity has grown, with the introductions of smoking bans in public places around the world. They are different from NRT in that they do not gradually reduce the amount of nicotine consumed, and so the ultimate aim is not necessarily to get the user free from nicotine addiction. Instead, some users find that they can make the switch to e-cigarettes and therefore stop smoking regular cigarettes, while others find that they help reduce the amount of regular cigarettes they smoke because they use the e-cigarettes periodically instead. Essentially they can be useful because they show the smoker that it's not the actual cigarette that's important to them, just the nicotine they contain. And of course they only contain nicotine – there are none of the other cancer-causing toxins and poisons that are in a conventional cigarette.

E-cigarettes help maintain all the same rituals and habitual behaviours around smoking – you can still go outside with your friends and have one, it looks and feels very similar to a regular cigarette and it has the added bonus of you being able to use them inside without the smell or risks of second-hand smoke to others. However, even though they are not tech-nically covered by many of the smoking bans because they do not emit smoke, some restaurants, hotels, train companies and airlines have already banned the use of e-cigarettes, citing various issues around complaints from other members of the public who confuse them for conventional cigarettes or express concern about the safety of passively inhaling the vapour.

Research published in the hugely respected medical journal *The Lancet* in September 2013, and presented at the European Respiratory Society, showed that e-cigarettes were at least as effective as patches in helping people stop smoking. Of those using e-cigarettes, 7.3 per cent had quit after six months, compared with 5.8 per cent using patches. After six months, 57 per cent of e-cigarette users had halved the number of tobacco cigarettes smoked each day compared with 41 per cent in those using patches. In the UK, 25 per cent of all attempts to kick the habit are made using e-cigarettes, making it the most popular quitting aid. Despite this, the response from the medical profession towards e-cigarettes has been lukewarm at best.

The authorities have several issues with e-cigarettes. Firstly, the industry is unregulated and therefore there are no laws governing exactly what is put inside them. Doctors and health campaigners argue that there's absolutely no guarantee of knowing what you are actually inhaling. There are also no rules around how they are sold or who they are sold to, meaning that, in theory, children could start buying them. There is also a wider issue they point to. They argue that e-cigarettes make smoking acceptable and visible again, which will promote it with youngsters. They see it as potentially a 'gateway' product that could lead people to experiment with the socially acceptable e-cigarettes and lead them to smoking tobacco.

I understand these concerns, but there is currently little evidence of this; instead, there is a growing evidence base that electronic cigarettes have considerable benefit in helping users quit smoking. The truth is that many smokers prefer e-cigarettes to the conventional nicotine replacement therapy offered by doctors, and the medical profession is notoriously slow to accept new or alternative options. I also suspect that some of the medical profession don't like the idea that people are taking quitting smoking into their own hands. I think some doctors resent the fact that people are now feeling empowered, have found something that they like and that works for them and are shunning the formal, official NHS-endorsed route to being smoke-free.

The other issue with e-cigarettes is that some people aren't necessarily using them to quit at all – they have simply switched to them as a safer alternative to smoking regular cigarettes and have no intention of stopping. It appears that this has enraged some of the critics, who, I suspect, have never smoked and are taking the hard-line purist stance that people shouldn't smoke at all – be it tobacco or nicotine vapour. Certainly no addiction is nice, but I really think that, from a pragmatic perspective, e-cigarettes are the lesser of two evils.

Legislation is now planned to regulate the sale and manu-facture of e-cigarettes across Europe, and it's only a matter of time before other countries around the world follow suit. It's all still quite early days for the e-cigarette, but, as yet, there's no clear evidence that they do any harm at all, and there's lots of evidence to suggest they can help people make a healthier choice and move away from conventional cigarettes. While the health impact of e-cigarettes has yet to be fully investigated, there is no doubt that they represent a *far* healthier option to regular smoking. It certainly seems a bit perverse that some in the medical profession want to see them banned because of unknown health risks, when the tobacco companies are allowed to continue to manufacture a product that has been demonstrated to be responsible for millions of deaths each year worldwide. In this regard, I fully support e-cigarettes.

So are they all good? Should you switch to them? There are a few issues. I used them for about a year before stopping smoking and I quite liked them. They are not the same as smoking a cigarette, despite what you might be told. It's difficult to gauge exactly how much you've 'smoked' because you don't extinguish them after a set number of puffs in the same way you do with a cigarette. Because of this, it's easy to keep puffing on them without thinking and actually ingest a very high level of nicotine without realising, until you suddenly feel very sick.

They also feel heavier in the hand and you have to suck much harder on them to inhale the vapour than you do with a tobacco cigarette. I found that, instead of holding them between my index and middle finger, as I would always do with a tobacco cigarette, they were too heavy for this to be comfortable, so I would have to hold them between my thumb and index finger, like a dart. I hadn't realised how something as simple as changing the way you hold something could have such a profound effect on the experience, but it just felt strange and alien to me. I was still smoking cigarettes at the time and only using them when I was somewhere I couldn't smoke, so perhaps if I'd switched entirely to them and ditched the cigarettes, I'd have soon got used to the new look and feel.

I've spoken to friends and patients who have used them about this and for some this was an issue too, while for others it wasn't. For me, I'd been smoking for so long and it had become so ritualised and habitual that any small change felt awkward and only reminded me that I wasn't 'properly' smoking. But, that aside, I liked their convenience, the fact I could use them inside if I wanted and the fact they didn't make me smell of stale smoke. They were a good way of silencing friends or family who disapproved of me smoking, especially in front of them and, I have to say, when I used them they did give me a brief feeling of relief that they weren't killing me.

Without this viable alternative to smoking, many people will continue to smoke cigarettes and surely no one wants this, so if you want to try them be my guest. However, you must realise that they do nothing except provide an alternative for getting nicotine into your system. They are not addressing your addiction to nicotine. Certainly they have the potential to help move you away from tobacco cigarettes and this can only be a good thing. But they do not dispel the myth that smoking or nicotine does anything for you. You're still an addict if you use e-cigarettes, and you're still wasting time and money and energy on something that is of absolutely no benefit to you whatsoever. Also, there's always the risk that if you continue to use e-cigarettes, you're still addicted to nicotine and therefore still highly vulnerable to relapsing back to tobacco.

So, my overall advice on e-cigarettes is: by all means try them if you want to, but continue to do the exercises in this book while you use them, as you still need to address the illusion, distortions and myths that are still present in your mind about the benefits of smoking.

ARE MILD AND MENTHOL CIGARETTES HEALTHIER?

I'm going to dispel a myth that exists around 'mild', 'low tar', 'light' or menthol cigarettes: they are absolutely not 'healthier' or in any way less damaging than regular cigarettes. People really struggle with this and it's not their fault – it just means that they have been victim to a very clever and enduring marketing campaign. To undo this, we need to go back over 60 years because these types of cigarettes have an interesting history.

In 1952, the magazine *Reader's Digest* ran a short article entitled 'Cancer by the Carton'. This two-page report became arguably the most important piece of consumer health journalism ever written. The impact of this article cannot be underestimated, and millions of people owe their lives to it. Its legacy stretches out far into the present day. In just a few hundred words, it alerted the public to growing concern within medical circles that smoking cigarettes was a risk factor for developing lung cancer. While this fact is now well accepted and forms the basis of countless public health campaigns and legislation, at the time of publication the public were largely ignorant of the increasing amount of medical evidence to suggest this link.

Before then, there had only been a handful of articles in the lay press suggesting that smoking was in any way bad for your health and, even then, they had largely been erroneous associations, linking it to tuberculosis or stunted growth. The tobacco industry had shrugged these off and continued to see soaring sales, thanks in no small part to its intense advertising campaigns, often fronted by doctors themselves. But the fallout from the *Reader's Digest* article resulted in the first decline in tobacco sales since the Second World War. It generated media interest in itself, and was suddenly being discussed around the globe. In fact, both my grandparents stopped smoking on the day they heard about the article. The outcry was so great that the Tobacco Industry Research Committee was forced to release a statement, saying: 'we believe our products are not injurious to health' and 'we always have and always will cooperate closely with those whose task it is to safeguard the public health'. But, while outwardly the committee attempted to provide a robust response to the article and the growing concern it generated among the public, privately it was panicking. Some committee members even reluctantly confessed that they had been researching the link themselves for several years.

Their main response to public health fears, though, was a very clever marketing campaign, the legacy of which is the 'light' or 'low tar' cigarette. First though, the tobacco companies started to promote filtered cigarettes. Rothmans quickly launched the first cigarette in Britain with a filtered tip, saying in adverts that it was 'the cigarette with the protection that so many smokers are seeking today'. Of course, the filter offers no protection against cancer or any of the other carcinogens in cigarettes. In reality, they were not a health device, but a marketing device. Indeed, privately, tobacco industry insiders referred to them as 'health image cigarettes'. However, it signalled the first loosening of the iron grip the tobacco companies had around the general public. For the first time in decades, they were on the back foot and they have never recovered.

When further research showed that, actually, adding a filter on to the cigarette did not help in any way, tobacco companies developed and heavily promoted the 'low tar' or 'light' cigarette. Once again, it was a marketing device, rather than any form of health device. It merely gave false reassurance that this product wasn't as bad as the others, when in fact, this is complete rubbish. Countless research has shown that this isn't the case – that smoking 'low tar' or 'light' cigarettes is just as bad for you. It's simply advertising that tells us otherwise.

Since regulation in the US has forced tobacco companies to make public their internal documents, there can now be no doubt that the industry deliberately sought to both maintain and expand its customer base by cynically manipulating smokers' health concerns. In other words, as people became more and more concerned about the health risks of smoking, the tobacco industry produced 'lighter' brands to try to convince the smoker they were making a 'healthier' choice and to keep them smoking.

But why, you might ask, do low tar cigarettes cause as much damage as regular cigarettes? The stroke of genius from the tobacco industry was that it seems to make sense that reducing the tar in a cigarette would result in a 'healthier' cigarette. But the problem is that there is a fundamental flaw in this thinking, and it's one that the tobacco industry tried to keep secret for a long time. If you look at the packet of a 'low tar' or 'light' box of cigarettes, you will indeed see that the reported levels of nicotine and tar are lower. These 'levels' are obtained by a special machine. What has now come to light is that, while it was always known that a machine could not mimic the exact smoking habits of a human, the tobacco industry had discovered how to design a cigarette that yielded low tar and nicotine levels when smoked by the machine, but considerably higher ones when smoked by a human. The tests also failed to take into account the 'compensation' that humans make when they smoke a 'light' cigarette. Humans, unlike a machine, are addicted to nicotine, so they unconsciously alter the way they inhale the smoke to ensure that they get the amount of nicotine they need to stave off cravings. For example, they smoke more 'intensively' by inhaling deeper into their lungs in order to get more smoke, and therefore more nicotine, with each puff. It's therefore downright misleading to claim that these cigarettes are 'light' or 'low tar'.

Because of this, legislation in many countries has recently been passed that bans the use of these terms because they gave false reassurance and the public wrongly thought these cigarettes would do less damage to their body. Instead, the tobacco companies have cleverly resorted to using colour coding on many of the packets, using pale colours or white to subtly suggest that they are not as 'strong' as regular cigarettes.

Likewise, menthol cigarettes are popular because many people wrongly believe that in some way they taste 'fresher' and therefore reduce the smell associated with regular cigarettes. They also confuse the idea of a menthol taste with being healthier in some way. It tastes a bit like toothpaste, so it must be all right, yeah? Absolutely not. Menthol cigarettes, as with 'light' or 'low tar' cigarettes, cause exactly the same damage as regular cigarettes.

All of these are marketing gimmicks designed to keep the smoker hooked and offer false reassurances that what they are doing is not killing them. It doesn't matter what brand you smoke, whether it tastes a bit minty or not, the damage done to your body is exactly the same.

Conclusion
The best thing you've ever done

Of all the things I have done and achieved in my life, stopping smoking is by far the best. It has given me back my life in a way that, while I was smoking, I did not think was possible. In fact, it has given me things back that I never even realised had been taken from me. After I stopped smoking, I felt like I'd been reborn. Everything was brighter and better. I no longer had the fear of the damage I was doing to myself looming over me, combined with the fear of having to stop and the unbearable tension this generated in my mind. I felt and looked better. But, more than anything, it showed me how powerful my mind was. It showed me that this seemingly enormous, overwhelming task could be achieved simply with the power of my mind. It showed me that by changing the way I thought, I could change my behaviour and achieve something I had spent most of my life believing was impossible. The buzz this gives you is like nothing else, and the sense of power and control it gives you in your life is something that I am so pleased I have discovered.

I do, of course, wish I had never smoked. I look back at the me who smoked and I feel pity for the person who felt so trapped and stuck that they had convinced themselves that they were in love with something that was slowly killing them. I feel anger and frustration at all the money I wasted on something that was totally pointless. But all the wishing in the world cannot turn back the clock and it's pointless spending time and energy trying. It is in the past now.

Throughout this book I have told you that smoking gives you nothing but that's not entirely true. Smoking did give me something and it can give it to you too. Or rather, it's the stopping smoking that gives you something. It gave me the opportunity to show to myself that I was stronger and more powerful than I had ever imagined. Even now, when I find myself doubting my abilities or facing something I think is daunting or impossible, I remind myself of this incredible achievement that I did entirely on my own with just me and my brain. Stopping smoking has given me self-confidence that I never knew possible. It has made me think that anything I want to achieve in life is now within my power. And you can have that feeling as well. All you have to do is stop smoking. Trust me, it's the best thing you will ever do.

Resources

If you've followed this book and done all the exercises, you should now be happily smoke-free. However, some people might want additional support and information. It's important that this information is accurate and impartial, so I've included a brief list of places you can go for more free information and advice.

The NHS has a lot of resources to help people who want to stop smoking. You can speak to your GP or pharmacist about stop-smoking programmes in your area if you want to try these in addition to this book, but the NHS also has some great resources on line:

http://www.nhs.uk/smokefree
https://quitnow.smokefree.nhs.uk

The charity Quit has a helpline and community programmes: http://www.quit.org.uk

There's also information about smoking and how to stop on the website of the charity Ash: http://www.ash.org.uk

For people in Scotland, there is a helpline for those thinking about stopping smoking: http://www.canstopsmoking.com/

Acknowledgements

I am indebted to Sam Jackson and Louise Francis for their help with writing this book. I am also very grateful to Jack Munnelly, Elly Cornwall, Celia Hayley, Claire Houghton-Price and Heather Holden-Brown for their advice and support. Thanks to Anne Lawrance and Lisa Highton for their encouragement with my writing. Sincere thanks also go to Rhiannon Doyle, Tasha Coccia-Clark, Jan Moir, Sarah McMahon, Sue Gibbs, Dean Thorpe, my mum and my sister who each, in their own way, helped me stop. Special thanks goes to Nick Deakin.

Index

abusive relationship, smoking as
    an 22–5
action 139–89
    avoiding triggers and breaking
        routines 165–7
    dealing with relapse 176–8
    detoxify your house 148
    exercise 14: recap 142
    exercise 15: visualise your first
        days as a non-smoker 146
    exercise 16: your quitting
        contract 156
    exercise 17: an expensive
        addiction 158
    exercise 18: progressive muscle
        relaxation 172–5
    getting rid of smoking
        paraphernalia 149–50
    money talks 157–9
    nicotine replacement therapies
        or medications 160–4
    preparing for action 141–2
    Q&As 179–89
    reducing before stopping
        151–2
    set a date 143–7
    tell a friend 153–4
    when triggers remain 168–9
    withdrawals 170–5
    write a contract 155–6

addiction, the basics of 41–75
    cravings 62–5
    exercise 3: the reasons to
        continue smoking 47, 94,
        101
    exercise 4: your one-day
        smoking diary 60–1
    exercise 5: the time you spend
        not smoking 64–5
    exercise 6: reasons to not smoke
        (your 'quit list') 68, 112
    exercise 7: imagine a smoke-free
        future 71–2, 91
    exercise 8: imagine a smoke-free
        past 74–5
    getting to grips with addiction
        57–61
    life without smoke 71–2
    mind, the power of the 66–8
    nicotine addiction, the myth of
        43–7
    physiological and psychological
        addiction 58, 59
    understanding the effects of
        nicotine 48–56
    why do people keep smoking?
        73–5
    willpower 69–70
ageing, smoking and 136
alveoli 48–9

ambivalence 111–12
    exercise 11: the golden tree 112
Ash 193

Beecher, Henry 67, 68
best thing you've ever done,
    stopping smoking as the
    191–2
boredom 33, 81–2, 169
brainwashing 38–9, 43

cancer:
    bladder cancer 134
    bowel cancer 134
    link between smoking and
        discovered 45–6, 185–6
    lung cancer 17–19, 126, 134
    mouth cancer 126, 134
    oesophageal cancer 126
    'one day' argument and 102
    pancreatic cancer 127
    physical benefits of not smoking
        and 134, 135
    stomach cancer 134
    throat cancer 126
    timeline of quitting and 126,
        127
    toxins and poisons in cigarettes
        and 175, 180
    willpower to give up smoking
        and diagnosis of 69
canstopsmoking.com 193
carbon monoxide 122–3, 126,
    138
CBT (cognitive behavioural
    therapy) 3–6, 20, 66, 99,
    151, 179
Champix 160, 161–2, 164
choice, smoking as a 19, 22
chronic obstructive pulmonary
    disease (COPD) 85–6
cilia 124–5, 126

circulation 122, 125, 134, 135,
    136
cognitive dissonance 79–80
cognitive shift 20
comforting, smoking as 115–16
concentration, smoking and 82–3,
    102–3
conditioning 118
counsellor, smoking-cessation 9,
    69
contract, write a quitting 155–6
cool, smoking and notions of
    31–2, 33, 34, 35, 37, 38–9,
    43, 144–5
coping strategy, smoking as a 19,
    115–17, 151
    exercise 12: new ways of coping
        116–17
cough:
    after giving up 124, 125
    cancer and persistent 18
    'smokers' 125
cravings:
    alleviating 170–1
    exercise 5: the time you spend
        not smoking 64–5
    length of 26, 62–5, 114, 122,
        171–2
    mild and menthol cigarettes and
        188
    nature of 62–5
    nicotine receptors and 52
    nicotine replacement therapy
        and 49
    progressive muscle relaxation
        (PMR) and 172–5
    reading this book and 9
    withdrawal and 170–5
cues, smoking 118–20
    exercise 13: thinking about your
        smoking diary 119–20

Dean, James 34
desire 9, 15, 46, 103, 108, 113–14
diabetes 126, 161
diary:
    thinking about your smoking diary (exercise 13) 119–20, 166
    your one-day smoking (exercise 4) 60–1, 82, 116, 118
dieting 128, 129, 132
dopamine 51, 53
drug addicts 6, 19, 58, 59, 97, 106, 109

electronic/e-cigarettes 179–85
emotionally charged associations 13, 33–4, 37, 38–9, 118, 120, 142, 166, 186
energy, effect of smoking upon levels of 137–8
enjoyment of smoking 1
    all-or-nothing thinking and 90
    as alleviation of withdrawal symptoms 73, 74, 84–5, 88, 102, 104
    concentration and 83, 102
    exercise 1: the reasons you smoke and 24–5
    genetics and 53, 54, 55
    parties and 90
    taste of cigarettes and 49–50
ex-smokers 15, 28–30, 46, 154, 163
exercise tolerance/fitness 16–17, 125–6, 130
exercises 7–8, 10–11, 100, 184–5, 193
    1: the reasons you smoke 24–5, 68, 79
    2: your smoking story 35–7

3: the reasons to continue smoking 47, 94, 101
4: your one-day smoking diary 60–1, 82, 116, 118
5: the time you spend *not* smoking 64–5
6: reasons to not smoke (your 'quit list') 68, 178
7: imagine a smoke-free future 71–2, 91, 146
8: imagine a smoke-free past 74–5
9: your own thinking errors 91–3, 131, 178
10: smoking on trial 94–6
11: the golden tree 112, 155
12: new ways of coping 116–17
13: thinking about your smoking diary 119–20, 166
14: recap 142
15: visualise your first days as a non-smoker 145
16: your quitting contract 156
17: an expensive addiction 158
18: progressive muscle relaxation 172–5
expensive addiction, an (exercise 17) 158
extroverts, smoking and 38

failure to stop smoking, previous 106–7
fertility 135–6
finances 19, 79, 110, 112, 121, 157–9, 184, 192
food, weight and cigarettes 128–9
friends:
    fear of losing 108
    telling you are planning to stop smoking 153–4

getting stuck 101–8

'I need it to concentrate'
102–3
'I'll lose my friends' 108
'I'll miss it too much' 104–5
'I've tried before and failed'
106–7
'It helps me cope' 105
'It makes me happy' 104
'It's not the right time' 101–2
'it's who I am' 105–6
'giving up' 26–7, 28
golden tree, the (exercise 11) 112,
155
GP 2, 8, 9, 18, 164, 193

happiness, smoking and 51, 104
heart disease 126, 127, 134
heroin 19, 44, 45, 58–9, 106,
109–10, 177
house, detoxify your 148

identity, smoking and 31–7,
38–9, 43, 105–6, 144–5
imagine a smoke-free future
(exercise 7) 71–2, 91, 146
imagine a smoke-free past
(exercise 8) 74–5
impotence 135

Lancet, The 181
language, cigarettes and 34, 39
lies we tell ourselves 79–88
'I enjoy smoking' 84–5
'I like the taste' 87–8
'I've got to die of something'
85–6
'If I stop smoking I'll gain
weight' 86–7
'It helps me concentrate' 82–3
'smoking helps alleviate
boredom' 81–2
'smoking helps me relax' 84

'smoking helps me when I'm
feeling stressed' 81
life without smoke 71–2
love of cigarettes/smoking 15–16,
18, 19, 20, 21, 22–5, 29, 33,
113, 142, 157, 162, 163, 192
lozenges 17, 160
lung cancer 17–18, 126, 134, 185
lungs:
cravings and 62
effects of nicotine and 48–9
electronic cigarettes 179
first cigarette and 16
'light' or 'low tar' cigarettes and
188
timeline of quitting and 124–6
physical benefits of not smoking
and 134, 138
withdrawals 171, 175

maladaptive coping strategy 115
medications, anti-smoking 8–9,
160–4
menstrual cycle 146–7
mild and menthol cigarettes 185–9
money, smoking and 19, 79, 112,
121, 157–9, 184, 192

NHS 8, 182, 193
nicotine, understanding the effects
of 48–56
different capacities for nicotine
and 54–6
dopamine release and 51
nicotine receptors and 50–2,
53–6
occasional smokers and 52–6
'receptor up-regulation' and
'down-regulation' 51–2
taste of cigarettes and 49–50
nicotine addiction:
difficulty of giving up 44

levels of nicotine in cigarettes and 44–5
the myth of 43–7
tobacco industry and 44–5
pharmaceutical industry and 45–6
nicotine replacement therapy and 45–7
nicotine gum/patches 160
 cravings and 49
 difficulty of giving up and 46
 efficacy of 15
 increase in amount of cigarettes smoked due to 17
 nicotine receptors and 59
 using this book in conjunction with 8
 willpower and 69
 see also nicotine replacement therapy (NRT)
nicotine receptors:
 nicotine addiction and 50–6, 57–8, 62–3, 123–4, 125, 126, 152, 161–2, 170, 176
 nicotine replacement medications and 161–2
 occasional smokers/different genetic types and 52–5
 'receptor down-regulation' 52, 123–4, 125, 126, 152, 170
 'receptor up-regulation' 51–2
 relapse and 176
 vary in their shape from person to person 53
 withdrawal and 170
nicotine replacement medications 8–9, 160–4
nicotine replacement therapy (NRT) 17, 45–7, 49, 160–4
 see also nicotine gum/patches
non-smoker not ex-smoker 28, 30

occasional smokers and 51–6, 177
'one day' argument 16, 69, 102, 141
opiate drugs 58–9, 63
other stop-smoking techniques, using this book with other 8–9

panicking, stop 1–2
paraphernalia, getting rid of smoking 149–50
peer pressure and the first time 31–7
 cool kids and 31–2, 33
 emotionally charged associations and 33–4
 exercise 2: your smoking story 35–7
 fear of effect upon character of stopping smoking 35
 idea of smoking and 32–3
 language of cigarettes and 34
 rebellious nature of smoking 34–5
 smoking as defining of your character 34
pharmaceutical industry 45–6
pharmacist 8, 160, 164, 180, 193
physical addiction to cigarettes 43, 77
 cravings and 62, 63, 114
 ex-smokers and 28
 mildness of 46
 mind and 68
 nicotine addiction and 28, 49
 nicotine replacement medications and 164
 opiates and 58, 59
physical benefits of not smoking 134–8
preparing for action 141

progressive muscle relaxation
(exercise 18) 172–5
psychological addiction to
cigarettes and 10
ex-smokers and 28–30
maladaptive coping strategy 115
nicotine replacement therapies
and 46–7, 163, 164
opiate drugs and 58–9, 109
reducing the amount you smoke
and 151
stages of change and 97–8
weight worries and 130, 131, 132

Q&As 179–89
'are mild and menthol cigarettes
healthier?' 185–9
'should you switch to electronic
cigarettes?' 179–85
Quit 193

reaction formation 29
Reader's Digest: 'Cancer by the
Carton' article 185–6
reasons to continue smoking:
exercise 3: reasons to continue
smoking 47, 94, 101
exercise 10: smoking on trial 95
vs reasons to quit 94–6
reasons to not smoke (your 'quit
list') (exercise 6) 68, 178
reasons you smoke (exercise 1)
24–5, 68, 79
recap (exercise 14) 142
red blood cells 122–3, 126, 138
reducing before stopping 151–2
relapse, dealing with:
contract and 155
dealing with 176–8
ex-smokers and 28
nicotine replacement
medications and 164

previous relapse preventing
attempt at quitting 106–7
reducing before stopping and
152
stages of change and 99
telling people you are quitting
and 153
weight worries and 128
withdrawal and 123
relaxation:
smoking and 19, 24, 25, 51, 84,
110
techniques 169, 172–5
resources 193
routines, breaking 165–7

scam, smoking as a 43
Scotland 193
Second World War, 1939–45 67,
68, 186
self-harm, smoking as 19–20
sex, need for and smoking 38
skin, smoking and 122, 126, 131,
136, 161
stages of change 97–100
action 99
contemplation 98
maintenance 99
pre-contemplation 98
preparation 98
story, your smoking (exercise 2)
35–7
stress 6, 10
alleviation of, smoking and
18–19, 20, 33, 55–6, 81, 90,
101–2, 105, 115,
116, 117, 119, 143, 151, 165
getting stuck and 101–2
setting a date for quitting and
143
smoking as an additional 105
as a trigger for smoking 165

stroke 85, 86, 126, 134, 135
Swartfigure, Andrew 32–3, 50

taste:
  of cigarettes 49–50, 87–8, 136,
    188–9
  menthol cigarettes 188–9
  timeline of quitting and sense of
    123
technique, the 3–4
teeth:
  blood circulation and 125, 136
  gums and 136–7
  teeth loss and 126
  timeline of quitting and 125, 126
  weight gain and 131
  whitening 159
thinking errors 89–93
  all-or-nothing thinking 90
  discounting the positive 90
  emotional reasoning 90
  exercise 9: your own thinking
    errors 91–3, 131, 178
  jumping to conclusions 91
  mental filter 90
  overgeneralisation 89
thoughts about smoking, your
    77–138
  ambivalence 111–12
  coping strategies 115–17
  cues 118–20
  desire 113–14
  getting stuck 101–8
  heroin and 109–10
  physical benefits of not smoking
    134–8
  reasons to continue vs reasons
    to quit 94–6
  the lies we tell ourselves 79–88
  the stages of change 97–100
  thinking errors 89–93
  timeline 121–7

weight worries 128–33
time you spend *not* smoking, the
    (exercise 5) 64–5
timeline (of quitting) 121–7
  after you've stopped for: 20
    minutes 122
  after you've stopped for: 2 hours
    122
  after you've stopped for: 8 hours
    122
  after you've stopped for: 12
    hours 122–3
  after you've stopped for: 24
    hours 123
  after you've stopped for: 48
    hours 123
  after you've stopped for: 72
    hours 123–4
  after you've stopped for: 4 days
    124–5
  after you've stopped for: 5–8
    days 125
  after you've stopped for: 10 days
    125
  after you've stopped for: 2 weeks
    125–6
  after you've stopped for: 4 weeks
    126
  after you've stopped for: 3
    months 126
  after you've stopped for: 9
    months 126
  after you've stopped for: 1 year
    126
  after you've stopped for: 5 years
    126
  after you've stopped for: 10
    years 126
  after you've stopped for: 13
    years 126
  after you've stopped for: 15
    years 127

timing of stopping smoking
101–2, 143–7
tobacco industry 57, 128
   advertising 34, 38, 186
   characteristics of smokers and
      33–5, 38–9, 43
   food, weight, cigarettes and
      128–9
   'health image cigarettes' and
      187–8
   language of cigarettes and 34
   nicotine addiction and 44–5, 57
   revelation of smoking's link to
      cancer and 186
trial, smoking on (exercise 10)
   94–6
triggers:
   avoiding 165–7
   cues 118–20
   detoxifying your house and 148,
      171, 178
   exercises and 10
   preparing for 139
   setting a date for quitting and
      143, 145
   smoking diary and 61, 119–20
   when they remain 168–9

visualise your first days as a non-
   smoker (exercise 15) 145

weight worries 86–7, 128–33
why do people keep smoking?
   73–4
why people smoke 13–40
   abusive relationship, smoking as
      an 22–5
   author's story of smoking and
      15–21
   brainwashing 38–9

ex-smokers are the worst 28–30
giving up 26–7
peer pressure and the first time
   31–7
willpower 41, 69–70
withdrawal:
   alleviating 170–5
   amount of time spent in 62–3,
      65
   as something to celebrate 47
   capacity for dealing with
      nicotine and 54
   concentration and 83, 102, 103
   cravings and 62, 63, 64
   decreasing nature of 58–9, 64,
      122–7, 170
   fear of prospect of 73, 79, 81,
      111, 170–5
   happiness and 104
   heroin/opiates and 58–9, 63
   imagining a smoke-free past and
      74
   mental filter and 90
   mildness of 62–3, 170
   nicotine receptors and 52, 54,
      58–9
   nicotine replacement
      medications and 161–2
   premenstrual tension and 147
   smoking as alleviation of 52, 54,
      58–9, 70, 73, 79, 81, 83, 85,
      88, 90, 102, 103, 104, 105,
      168, 170–5
   stress and 81
   timeline of after quitting 122–7
   way we think about smoking
      and 43–4
   what it really is 3

Zyban 160–1, 164